Once Upon a Challenge:
Hearing is Believing

———————————— **Nancy L. Burns** ————————————

iUniverse, Inc.
New York   Bloomington

Once Upon a Challenge: Hearing is Believing

iUniverse books may be ordered through booksellers or by contacting:

iUniverse
1663 Liberty Drive
Bloomington, IN 47403
www.iuniverse.com
1-800-Authors (1-800-288-4677)

*Because of the dynamic nature of the Internet, any Web addresses or links contained in this
book may have changed since publication and may no longer be valid. The views expressed
in this work are solely those of the author and do not necessarily reflect the views of the
publisher, and the publisher hereby disclaims any responsibility for them.*

ISBN: 978-1-4401-5409-6 (pbk)
ISBN: 978-1-4401-5408-9 (cloth)
ISBN: 978-1-4401-5410-2 (ebook)

Printed in the United States of America

iUniverse rev. date: 7/20/09

Epilogue

"Regardless of how small or how enormous problems may appear to be, for every problem there is a solution.

"The real tragedy in my life has never been my lack of vision. The tragedy has been society's attitude toward my blindness."

Nancy Burns

CONTENTS

PREFACE

A message of love and caring and a desire to enlighten is contained within the pages of this book. I have shared many of my own real-life experiences in order to bring credibility to this message. Those of us who have been labeled as different must wear this label as a result of misconceptions and inaccurate stereotypes on the part of the general public. If we, the blind population, dare to speak out or attempt to correct these false notions, we are sometimes called rude or uppity. I know this; for as a wife, mother and a professional woman who happens to be blind, I am frequently the recipient of such demeaning responses.

Everyone experiences difficulties from time to time. The manner in which we choose to live with these challenges is the key to success. There are those who choose to maximize problems or to live as others perceive them. Existing within these imagined guidelines is unproductive, creates unhappiness and is a waste of gifts and talents.

Adversity can be humbling; but it can also be one of our most powerful teachers. I believe that there is a reason for all things. I also believe that for every problem there is a solution. As I relate some of these true experiences perhaps you will take the time to reevaluate some of the belief systems you may hold. I also hope to entertain you along the way as I attempt to unravel some of the misconceptions about blindness that are so tightly woven into the very fabric of our society.

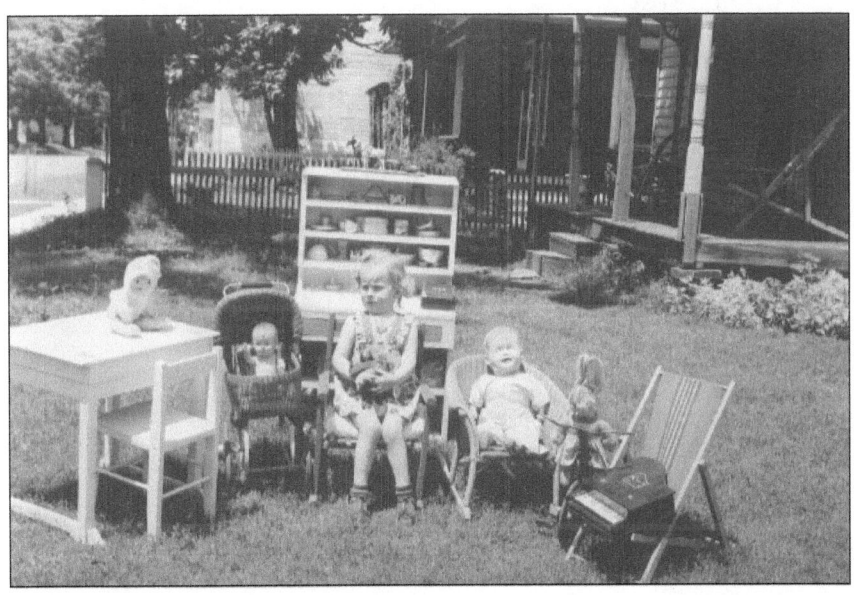

Tea time

Life is fairly uncomplicated for most eleven-year-old girls. Major concerns generally revolve around such things as "What shall I wear to school today?" "How fast can I get through this math assignment?" And "How can I meet that cute guy I see in the cafeteria everyday?"

And so it was for one tall, skinny sixth grader in the mid west. That is, until that terrible, fateful day when her life was turned completely upside down. She picked up a shiny object and became the innocent victim of a tragic circumstance. Some sort of explosive had been carelessly left behind and it did what it had been intended to do—but at the wrong time and in the wrong place. In one terrible instant her life was forever changed. She was blind, she was devastated.

I know all of this for I was that eleven-year-old girl. The world as I had known it for those eleven years was suddenly and tragically gone and would never be the same.

CHAPTER ONE

I Remember

For many years after this trauma and my resulting blindness, I simply adjusted to what was, and tried to understand why. I had no one around to reassure and to encourage me. I somehow muddled through and learned many things during my years of muddling. No one should have to go through such life experiences without finding a mentor or an advocate for guidance. I felt alone. I felt different. I was struggling to understand my new position in the world around me.

After my injury I spent several weeks in the hospital with both eyes bandaged. I just wanted someone to hold me and to tell me it would be okay. This never happened. I remember the day I came home from the hospital and how awkward and uncomfortable it was for everyone, including me. My sister and I were living with our grandparents and I was completely familiar with those surroundings. I could navigate fairly well through the house until someone left a chair or other obstacle in my way. It would take time for me to comfortably move through the house. I was always concerned that I would bump into something and look foolish. My mother, an extremely critical person, required perfection at all times from her daughters. How could I resolve this issue now that I was no longer perfect in her eyes?

This took place in the late 1940s and apparently there were no counseling services available. My family members did not know how to deal with this tragedy so they just didn't. I can't remember my mother ever saying the word "blind". My injury was simply referred to by her and others as "your accident" as if I had been the guilty perpetrator of this senseless and horrific act. I carried this erroneous guilt around with me for many years. It took some years of maturing and more than a few hours of gut-wrenching therapy to work through all of this.

My mother, Pauline, was one of two siblings born in rural Missouri. Her parents were divorced when she was very young and she was never allowed to know her father. She and her brother LeeRoy were moved around a lot as her single Mom took different jobs in order to support the family. When Mother was ten years old, her mother (my grandmother), met the man who would become my mother's step-father. Pauline became very fond of this man. He worked as a meat cutter, farmer, and eventually owned a feed store in a small town in Missouri. They were conservative, hard working, Southern Baptists.

Much of Mother's life is a mystery as she rarely shared many of her past experiences. It is not known why Mother became very controlling and very critical. We just know that it happened. Her constant criticism caused me to become somewhat sensitive to most criticism, constructive or otherwise. Mom spoke volumes with her facial expressions and body language. After losing my sight, my sister and I often joked about the fact that I could no longer see some of her disapproving facial expressions, but I knew they were there.

As did her mother, our mother divorced when my sister and I were very young and we were never allowed to know our father. As an adult I chose to connect with him which I did. Tragically, soon after we reconnected he died of a massive heart attack while only in his early 50's.

Years before my vision loss, an event had taken place that would eventually impact the philosophy and direction of my life. This event was the formation of the National Federation of the Blind (NFB)[1] by a blind visionary by the name of Dr. Jacobus tenBroek. It would be many years before I would find, and involve myself, in this positive-oriented organization. But it did eventually happen and I have learned volumes about living as a successful and "normal" blind person. My developing philosophy of life was in harmony with that of this nation-wide organization of blind people.

I know beyond the shadow of a doubt the reason for my existence on planet Earth. The Universe gives each of us challenges. It also provides us opportunities with which to meet these challenges and to learn and grow as a result of them. I knew, even as a young child, that I was the same person I had always been. The rest of the world, however, did not see it that way. The real tragedy in my life has never been my lack of eyesight. The real tragedy has been the false attitudes and misconceptions of society. What a disservice society causes in the process of labeling. Labels are mostly based on inaccurate stereotypes. These stereotypes are self-perpetuating and harmful. They are not the essence of a person. It is the soul or spirit that defines a human being.

Amazingly enough, these misconceptions are picked up and held by children at a relatively early age. Perhaps that was the reason for my own concern and confusion when I lost my sight. I felt that my life as an average, "normal" (whatever that is) kid was gone, and I had no idea what I could or could not do as a blind child. Little by little I began to comprehend the importance of my other senses.

With my vivid visual recall, I remembered every detail of Grandma's house. I pictured the dark wooden furniture in the dining room, including the large round dinner table. It was always covered with a crocheted tablecloth and in the middle was placed an antique footed fruit bowl. It rarely contained fruit but usually a variety of items such as pens, pencils and paper clips. If I barely touched the tablecloth I knew exactly where I was standing. My feet became accustomed to noticing the different textures between the hardwood floor of the dining room and that of the linoleum covering on the kitchen floor. Standing in the kitchen doorway, I could picture the built-in pantry in the far corner of the room. The sink was to my left and the more casual kitchen table, located in the middle of the room, was always covered with a freshly laundered cotton flowered tablecloth. The door to the back porch was beyond the table. If I stepped outside onto the porch my swing was still hanging there. I could manage that. Piece of cake!

My injury left me with scar tissue and other complications which finally caused a total loss of vision. Surgery after painful surgery met with little or no success. I struggled to return to the school I had attended. I could not keep up with the reading even with my grandmother's desire to help. An instructor from a training program came to the house. She wanted to teach me to read and write

Braille. My grandmother told her that I would not need to learn Braille as she was praying for me and the doctor was going to "fix" my eyes. This was, of course, part of my family's denial. The admission that I needed to learn to read Braille would be a clear acknowledgment that I was indeed blind.

During my frequent trips to the ophthalmologist, a sort of bonding occurred. On the day he felt the need to admit there was nothing more he could do, he presented me with a gift. He knew that I loved music and gave me an album of my favorite songs. I am sure that he believed I was doomed to a life of unhappiness and dependence. I don't often think about those confusing years following my vision loss. In reflecting back, I am not sure how this happened but apparently I simply was able to re-evaluate my life circumstances on nearly a daily basis. I am very thankful for those eleven years when I had perfect vision. I must have been a very observant child as I still picture things and places vividly in my imagination. I remember colors, at least the basic ones. It is sometimes hard for me to picture the different shades of colors that exist today. I take a great deal of pride in my wardrobe and will not step out of the house if I believe I am not perfectly coordinated. I know what colors I like and I enjoy keeping up with the fashion trends.

To this day I remember Robert Louis Stevenson's

poem, "The Swing" with the picture of a swing soaring over a garden wall. I can picture our tiny house in a residential area of southern Missouri. I remember the golden-brown-spotted tiger lilies in my grandmother's flower garden. I remember peeling an orange and pulling the white stuff from each section. I can still picture my grandmother sitting on the front porch crocheting something beautiful.

Sometimes I am not even sure if I had really seen something or if I am just able to picture it in my mind's eye. For example, I was recently discussing this with my sister. She asked me if I had ever seen an elephant. I quickly answered yes, and then had to stop and think about it. I certainly know what an elephant looks like from pictures, but I am not sure that I had ever really seen one as a child. I had never given this question any thought until my sister brought it up. I am still not sure if I really did see an elephant. My sister jokingly ended the conversation by saying that elephants sort of resemble a moving apartment building.

I do remember seeing a pebble thrown into a pond and watching the ripples. I remember being totally intrigued while watching a tiny hummingbird as it appeared to sit in mid air. I remember looking at the perfect rows of corn growing in a huge field, and I remember picking blackberries from the thorny bushes. I remember looking down a railroad track and seeing how the tracks appeared to come together in the distance. I remember walking along a white picket fence and looking down at the green velvety grass below.

I have lived most of my life as a blind woman. I am grateful for those eleven years when I experienced the world visually. My experiences today are no less wonderful or less exciting or less beautiful now that I am blind. My other senses have not improved, as is commonly believed; I have simply learned to utilize them to the max. As I take in the delicate fragrance of a rose from my husband's favorite coral rose-bush, I am able to enjoy this scent as well as see the rose in my mind's eye.

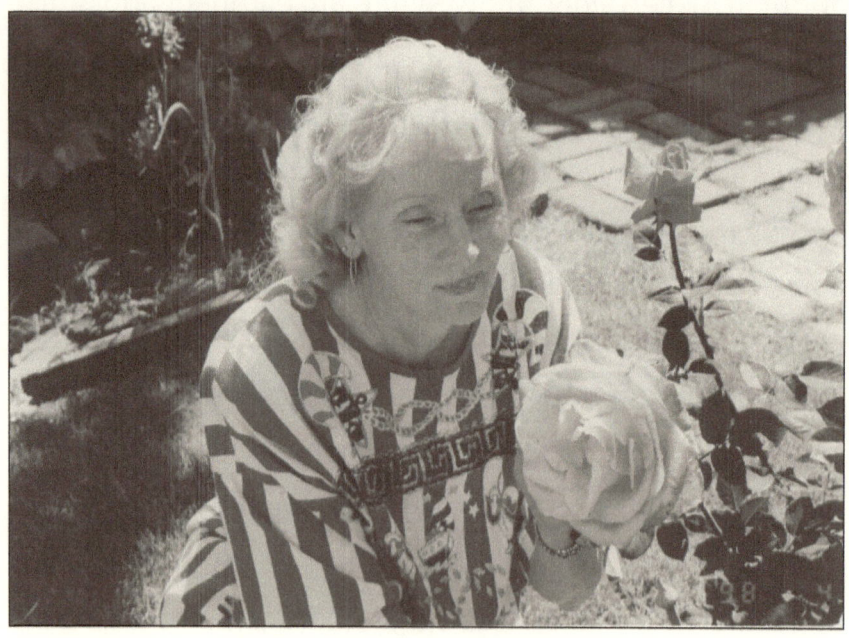

Don told me, "See what God and I have made for you."

CHAPTER TWO

Suzy

My vision loss occurred just a few months into my sixth grade year of school. The news of my injury and resulting blindness sent shock waves through the small Missouri town. Concepts relating to the equal rights for people with disabilities were non-existent. Legislation such as, the Americans with Disabilities Act[2], was still decades away. I suppose it is reasonable to understand the inability of most of my classmates to relate to me as I was now forced to assume a new role in society. I was neither brighter nor less bright now that I no longer experienced the world visually. I knew I was the same little kid with the same strengths and the same weaknesses. It did change the way in which I would perceive the world and sometimes the way in which I would now be perceived by the world.

There was one exception to this evasive behavior which most students exhibited. This one shining star, this one invaluable exception was my friend Suzy. I was able to maintain the friendship with Sue which had somehow survived the trauma of my vision loss.

She was caring and fun. We walked to the nearby soda fountain where we sipped cherry sodas and giggled. As most teenagers would do, we bought romance magazines. Suzy would read story after story until her eyes were nearly crossed. Grandma usually had a pitcher of lemonade or iced tea for us to enjoy while we discussed our next plan of action.

It was great when Sue got her car and she could drive us to her home which was in a rather rural area. Her family was as accepting of me as she was. On an overnight sleep-over we spied on her older sister who was returning home from an evening out with her boyfriend. We just did normal stuff and she helped me to regain the feeling that I might once again be able to have meaningful friendships. Over the years I have been blessed with many other "Suzys" in my life. A neighbor would drive me to the doctor's office if I had a sick child. Another might pick up a prescription or a loaf of bread. I made it a point to repay these most appreciated acts of kindness if only with a home-baked cookie and a cup of coffee. I have never wanted to be considered a burden to anyone and enjoyed the opportunity to pay back. Life would be greatly improved if there were more "Suzys" in the world.

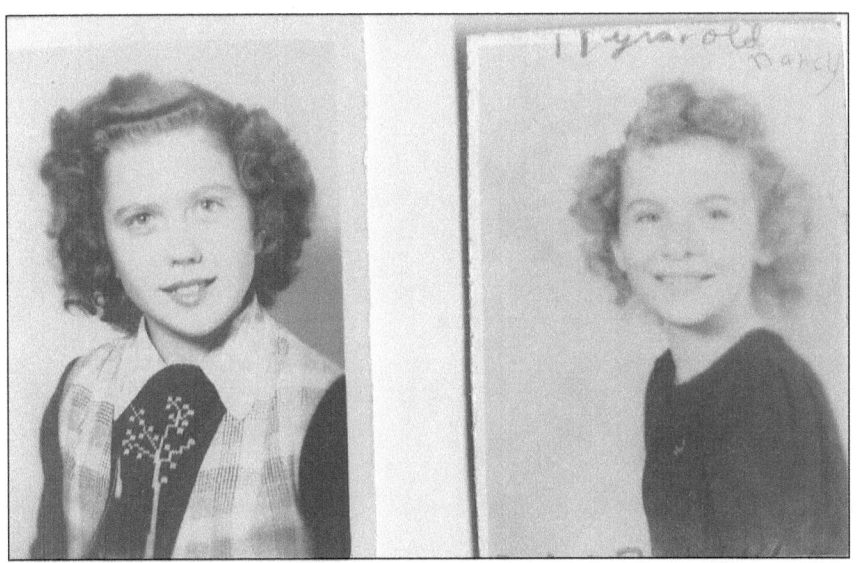

Suzy and Nancy

CHAPTER THREE

The Sixth Sense

As I matured and adjusted to my blindness, life was still fascinating although sometimes a little more challenging. I began to learn that there were some skills that I would need to be successful. Literacy, whether print or Braille, was essential and I would conquer that. I needed to be able to get from point A to point B independently. After a short experience with a guide dog, I opted for the white cane. I found it more convenient to come home and park my cane behind the door rather than having to feed, groom, and pick up after a dog. It took some time and training but I soon became confident as a blind traveler and have put this skill to use all over the U.S. and even outside the country.

There has been extensive discussion, particularly

in literature, about the "sixth sense." Contrary to popular belief my other senses did not improve after my vision loss but I certainly did learn to rely on them more. My sense of smell, for example, was not suddenly enhanced I just became more aware of the surrounding smells. This became somewhat annoying to my mother as she said I could smell a doughnut shop from a mile away. Needless to say, doughnuts were a popular item for me. I am also a fan of chocolate—just about anything chocolate works. As I was shopping in a grocery store one day I began to smell the wonderful aroma of something chocolate being baked. I was soon thinking about brownies and made my way to the bakery. I was already making my decision. Would it be frosted, plain, with pecans, or without? The possibilities were almost endless. I approached the counter and asked "What kind of brownies do you have"? There was a long pause and the woman behind the counter finally responded "square."

And then there is the sense of hearing, probably the most important of my senses. The best news of all is that music has always been important to me and guess what—music still sounded the same. No better; no worse. During my high school and college years I preferred rock and roll. My taste has changed to include many differing kinds of music, but my preference has gradually moved toward country western. Give me a Texas two-step or a waltz (with a little classic rock thrown in for good measure) and I am a happy dancer. But back to my basic skills, as I travel down a sidewalk I concentrate on the flow of traffic to know where and when to cross a street. I must say that it is becoming more challenging as drivers seem to ignore signals and appear less concerned about pedestrian safety. Hearing became invaluable as I raised my two sons. In addition to keeping track of their whereabouts, I could identify any toy or other object they picked up simply by the sound it made.

As I travel extensively, my hearing helps me to navigate through many situations including the ladies room. Recently I was in an airport restroom and a helpful woman gave me some great verbal instructions as I headed toward the sink. She told me that the sink was straight ahead, the soap was on the right and paper towels were on the left. As I washed my hands she explained that her father was blind and she knew he appreciated verbal directions. After I dropped the towel into the trash container she told me the exit was a few steps ahead and then to the left. I was pleasantly surprised by all of this and as I made the left turn I turned around, waved, and said "You're great. Thanks." On another occasion, my husband Don and I were waiting in a train station. A woman seated nearby said to Don "Tell her that her shoe is untied." I smiled (with some effort) and told her it was okay to tell me since I am the one who ties them. Another rather amusing incident took place as I was traveling alone from Los Angeles to New York. As we landed at Kennedy Airport the flight attendant asked if I needed any assistance. I said it would be helpful if someone could just walk with me to the shuttle area. As I left the plane, someone met me and walked with me to ground transportation. While approaching the shuttle, the driver asked the person accompanying me "Does she need a wheelchair"? I did a little dance and advised the man that my feet worked just fine and that it was my eyes that did not work so well.

I have addressed the issues of smell and taste in the doughnut-brownie incidents. My hearing, although no better than yours, is my constant aid. My sense of touch allows me to read Braille and to identify just about anything from my favorite red velour jacket to the variety of spices, utensils, and other items in my kitchen. So what about this sixth sense? Perhaps it has become apparent to you, as it has to me, that the sixth sense is most obviously a sense of humor. My sense of humor keeps me on track through such incidents as the shoe lacing advisor and shuttle driver incidents. Whether experiencing any disability or not, isn't a sense of humor a fabulous gift? Laughter is just good for the soul.

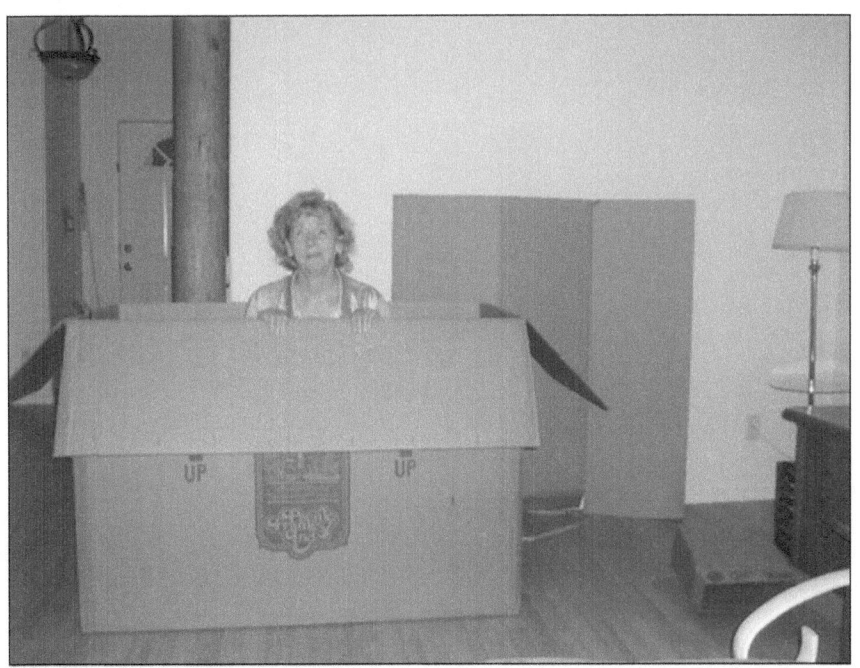

The Empty Furniture Carton Was Too Much to Resist

CHAPTER FOUR

This White Cane

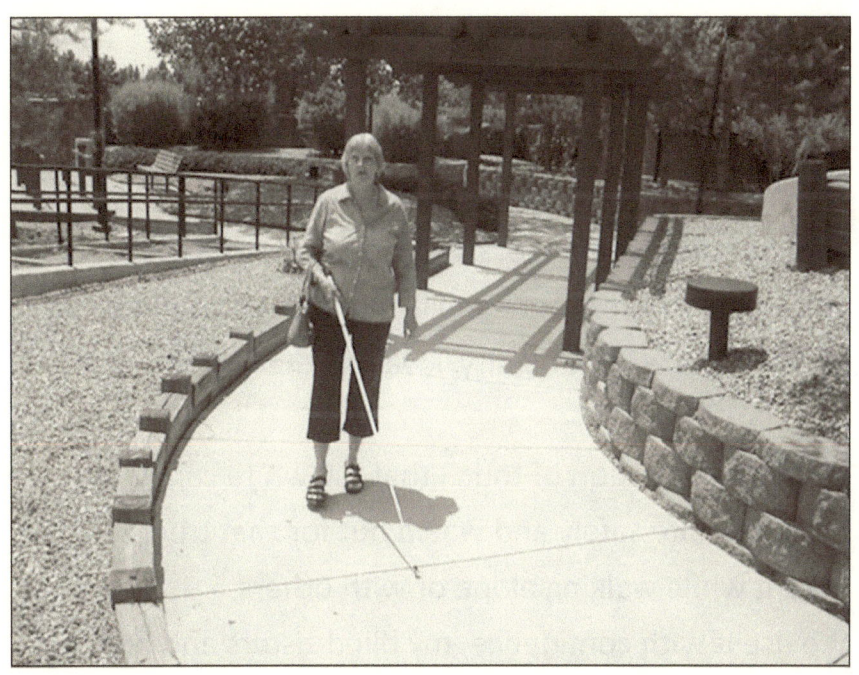

My Independence

The following poem was inspired by a sermon given by Pastor David Snyman, Paradise Hills United Methodist Church, Albuquerque, New Mexico (2008). He spoke on the pitfalls of judging others. Upon realizing how often I have been the recipient of such judgment, the words to this poem simply rushed into my mind and the poem was finished that very day.

This White Cane

When you see me approach with my white cane in hand
Are you quick to judge and not to understand
That I am not someone who needs pity and care
This cane will find doorways, a curb or a stair.

This is my independence—a valuable tool
That got me to neighbors and stores and to school
When my children were small and needed a guide.
I walked there with dignity, I walked there with pride.

With the extension of touch that my white cane gives me
I can navigate safely and watch out for that tree.
I use it while walking alone or with others,
We use it with confidence, my blind sisters and brothers.

I took buses to work—I have stories to tell,
I saved money for a trip and it went quite well.
I traveled to London to visit a friend,
I went shopping at Harrods, I had money to spend.

This white cane and I have traveled coast to coast,
This message is to teach; it is not meant to boast.

And now when you see us with white cane in hand
Please try not to label, just try to understand
That we do not want pity—just open your mind
And help us to change what it means to be blind.

Chapter Five

The World of Mentoring and Advocacy

As I indicated earlier, my sudden loss of sight was traumatic at best. Initially I had a tiny bit of vision and I tried to go back to the school that I had been attending. It just did not work. I could not see the blackboard nor could I keep up with the reading. I missed over a year of school with all of this and was finally sent to the Missouri School for the Blind in St. Louis.[3]

The school was 300 miles from home and was a residential school. Students from all over the state attended. On my initial visit my mother and I met the staff and toured the facilities. She left for home and there I was now in a completely unfamiliar building. I had no skills and no self confidence. Once again, I was feeling very alone and very overwhelmed. I had never seen this large building before so I had no mental images to assist in my orientation. The dormitory was a long, rectangular room with beds on both sides and metal lockers against the wall at the head of each bed. I learned to walk down the long aisle with my hand barely touching the foot of each bed. My bed and locker were in the very back of this room. My 16 roommates seemed to be pretty "normal," whatever that is. They were doing the things I was not sure I could ever do again. They maneuvered through the long hallways and ran up and down the stairs. They roller skated, played games and studied with the use of Braille. I began to think that I just might be okay after all. These diverse roommates were friendly and helpful and I soon learned my way around the large campus. With each new accomplishment came the return of some of my self confidence. These young girls made a tremendous impact on my life and helped me to focus on what I could do rather than on what I believed I could no longer do.

The academic standards of this school were very high. I was soon learning everything from literature to algebra in Braille. The Braille code was easy enough for me to learn but picking up speed was the trick. It was taking me longer to get my homework completed but I could now function in school independently. We were also given tasks to perform in our spare time such as drying dishes in the huge kitchens or over-seeing the smaller children while their house mothers went to dinner. Home economics and physical education were also a part of the curriculum. It was a fairly well-rounded educational system. This gigantic learning experience was truly the first step toward my independence as a blind woman. I spent about four years at this school and these were four of the most important years of my life. This is where I learned to live in my circumstances. This is where I began to learn that there were others in my situation – others with whom I could relate. We played cards and talked about boys as I had done as a sighted kid. Saturday nights were date nights. Sometimes it was popcorn and bingo; and about once a month there would be a dance. The other good news is that there were teachers and staff members who believed in us and who had high expectations of us. I had just come from an environment in which no one had any confidence in the fact that I might someday be an independent, successful person as my sighted peers would be.

It was in this setting where I learned (although I didn't recognize it as such at the time) that I had advocacy pulsing through my veins. I don't know the origin or the reason for this aspect of my personality—it just happened. In each dorm of 15 or 16 girls there was a supervisor known as a house mother. My house mother, we'll call her Mrs. Brown, seemed nice enough at first but we soon became at odds with each other. We all looked forward to receiving letters and packages from home. My grandma sent wonderful care packages of homemade cookies on a routine basis. Other friends and family members would send goodies. Mrs. Brown would let me open my cherished box but then it disappeared into her closet. When I wanted something from it I would have to go and ask her for my package. I began to notice that the goodies sometimes rapidly disappeared. I started keeping close track and also compared notes with other girls who were experiencing the same phenomenon.

The housemothers went to dinner half an hour before the rest of us and for that short time we were left alone in the dorm. On one occasion I gathered up three or four other girls and we visited the principal's office with our concerns. We were all nervous but we did it. We had a sympathetic session with the principal but, of course, he maintained a neutral view throughout our visit. During the next few weeks, we noticed a change in tactics with our relished gifts from home. We were allowed to keep them in our lockers as long as they remained wrapped. I have recognized advocacy as an important aspect of my character only in retrospect. At the time, I just believed that we were being treated badly and that we should do something about it. I suppose this was the birthplace of my concern and my passion for individual rights, regardless of our circumstances.

Just as I was getting a handle on this blindness thing another huge challenge presented itself. My family was moving to California. I was now comfortable in school. I was getting good grades and had a boyfriend—the best-looking, and most popular guy in my class. My sister was in elementary school and she was not looking forward to attending a large metropolitan school. I assumed that I would be attending a residential school in California but this was not to be the case. Residential schools were becoming crowded and the practice of main-streaming was now very popular. This meant that I could stay at home and attend a regular public school; but it was in Los Angeles and it was big. I was again looking at a new experience; but I was up for the challenge.

The campus was huge with a student enrollment of over one thousand. In one of the buildings there was a section called the resource room. Blind students could bring homework or tests to this room where a teacher aid would provide reading. No more Braille books. I could, however, take notes with my slate and stylus. There were eight or ten other blind students and we were bused in from the surrounding area.

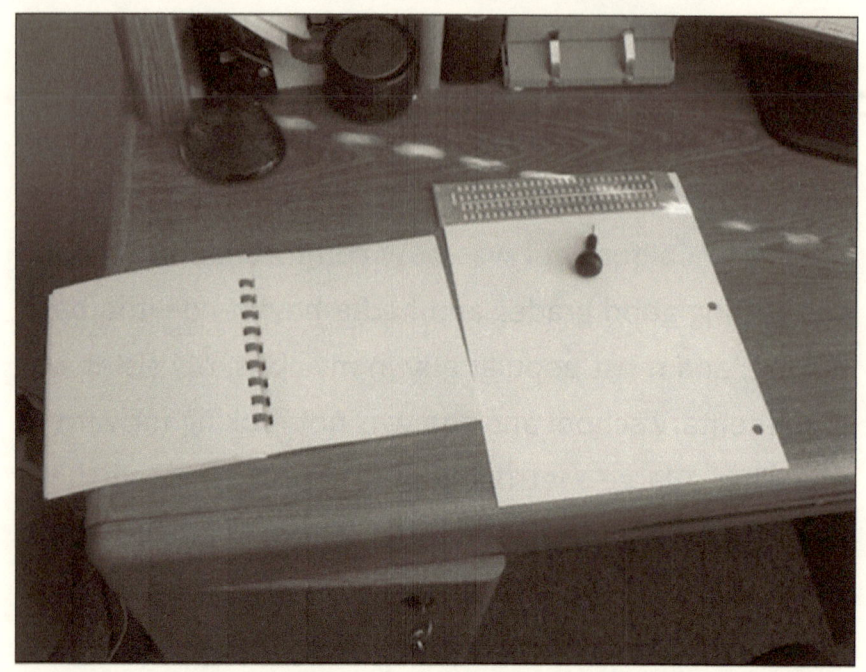

Slate and Stylus Used for Writing Braille. Numerous electronic note-taking devices are now available for Braille readers.

The teacher in charge of the resource room was a wonderful woman who happened to be blind. Mrs. G. was one of the most important mentors in my life. She had much more confidence in me than I had in myself. She told me that I should take college prerequisites but I argued that I did not like geometry and some of that other stuff. She won and I managed to take all of the necessary courses in order to go to UCLA.

Although at first the thought of attending this large public high school was very intimidating, it was truly a positive and important step in my educational process. It became a challenging, but worthwhile, transition from the segregated school for the blind to the bigger world of sighted people.

Mrs. G. was also instrumental in introducing me to the National Federation of the Blind (NFB). This is an organization *of* the blind not *for* the blind. I met and mingled with successful blind people from all walks of life. The world was opening up to me even more. It was in this organization that I met a counselor, also blind, who told me "it is respectable to be blind." I met him during my college years and was not quite convinced at that time in my life that this was indeed the truth. I have learned it to be the truth and give so much credit to those first blind boys and girls I met in St. Louis and then to the blind adults I met later in life. During my college years I began to meet high-functioning, motivated blind students who were pursuing all kinds of careers that I had never imagined could be possible. Wow! I had discovered a virtual treasure trove of mind-expanding ideas and possibilities. Life was challenging, but life was good.

From my college years and beyond I found enormous support from my blind sisters and brothers. If I ran into a problem, with most anything from student issues to "how to" issues I could always find someone with the answer. I was not aware that there were blind people from nearly every walk of life including electricians, teachers, lawyers and mechanics. My awareness of my own possibilities in life was unfolding.

The NFB is a people-driven organization of blind, and interested sighted individuals who work for common goals. The mission of the NFB is to bring equality in all areas of life to people who are blind or visually impaired. Much of my philosophy of life is based on my experiences with this dynamic and caring organization. I have devoted much time and energy toward working with the NFB which is organized in every state, Washington D.C. and Puerto Rico, with headquarters in Baltimore, Maryland. I served on the Board of Directors for many years and was later elected president of the NFB of California. After my retirement from my position as a vocational counselor with the California Department of Rehabilitation, I served for six years as NFBC President. This was a volunteer position as no NFB officers are salaried. It was a full-time position based on love and caring for what I was doing. It was wonderful to have the experience of meeting a blind or visually impaired person who was convinced that his/her life as an independent person was over and then to see that person gradually gain self confidence through the process of mixing and mingling with other blind people. That was my paycheck.

On one occasion, a woman contacted me about

her blind brother in Japan. He recently lost most of his sight and was traveling to the U.S. and wanted to talk with some blind people here. He had lost his sight from retinitis pigmentosa[4]. I set up an appointment with the young blind man, his wife and sister and a member of the NFB who had lost his sight as a result of the same eye disease. His wife mostly cried during the entire meeting. I showed him some basics such as how to fold and identify paper money. He was shown some technology and we discussed training with a white cane.

At times, there were some difficulties as a result of the language barrier. The blind man spoke little English but his sister was able to interpret. Apparently the message of hope took as I received encouraging reports from the sister who had now become a member of the NFB and volunteer in the busy California office. He was receiving training to get him back to work and he now called his white cane his "magic stick." Those are the kinds of successes that kept me going.

I never considered myself to be a political person; I operated strongly from the passion I felt about my responsibilities as president of this organization. It was my pleasure to work with the twenty local chapters within the state. I organized and presented hundreds of workshops and seminars with subjects ranging from leadership techniques, motivation, and Braille advocacy to chapter strengthening. As within every organization, at least in my experience, there are usually a handful of people who do most of the work while others sit back and complain or do nothing. After my six years as president, I was ready to again retire, but with the feeling that I had accomplished much, created new programs, and had improved the lives of blind and visually impaired people along the way[5].

The outreach programs and services of this organization are wonderful. We work with seniors who are experiencing vision loss, provide scholarships for blind students, provide mentoring programs for any blind or visually impaired person. Of particular importance to me, perhaps due to my own childhood experiences, is the program which works with parents of blind children. All too often loving and well-meaning parents unwittingly create an environment based on low expectations. Such parents often hold inaccurate and harmful stereotypes about blindness. Blind children cannot reach their potential growth and development if the parents themselves do not hold positive expectations. Age-appropriate activities such as running, swinging, exploring and playing with other children are sometimes denied the blind child. Such activities are invaluable. They are invaluable to these parents and for the success of the lives of the blind children they touch. As with all things, knowledge is the key.

One of the programs I initiated was called Beginning Braille for Parents[6]. As sighted children begin to learn to read, they live in a print rich environment. This is not so with a blind child. Quite often the parents do not know Braille and are unable to assist their blind child with homework. The exceptions to this rule are extremely rare. Usually by the end of a day-long seminar parents were able to read and write some very basic Braille. Parents would write love notes to their children or messages such as "take out the trash" and were excited about their new skills.

I take a great deal of satisfaction from my work with the Federation. I also know that I have a better quality of life because of this organization. It is the perfect example of giving back to others the gifts they have given to you.[7]

CHAPTER SIX

Of Toilets and Garbage Disposals

When it comes to things around the house, I have always been fairly mechanically inclined. I am a good problem solver so I suppose this is helpful. All of this is simply to say that I don't normally back away from challenges. So when my husband (at that time) and I were asked to manage a large apartment complex in Hollywood, I was not intimidated by this responsibility.

We were newlyweds and thought the prospect of free rent in return for our services would help us to stockpile some funds. The owners were close friends of a friend. They agreed to take care of any major problems if we would collect rent and troubleshoot minor problems.

I must say that I did not feel readily accepted and for a couple of reasons. The majority of the tenants were older, retired people. Apparently the previous apartment managers were also older, retired people. Now we were taking over as a young newlywed couple, and one of us was totally blind. My husband was a social worker and went off to work early each day. As I got to know the tenants a little better I slowly gained their confidence. A couple of incidents in particular helped to move this process along. One morning Mrs. B. called and said her toilet would not stop running. I assured her that I would be right there. As I collected my cane, and a handful of courage, I worked my way to her apartment. She lived in the rear of the complex on the second level. I had never been in her apartment. Before knocking I paused slightly to regroup. She opened the door quickly. I stepped inside and could immediately hear the running water from the toilet. Using my cane, I carefully navigated around her coffee table and went directly into the bathroom. I checked to make sure nothing was on the back of the toilet and lifted the lid, laying it on the seat. I reached inside and found that the "whatever it is called" had not closed and the water in the tank was a continuous flow. I moved the "whatever" over and closed the opening. Once the tank was filled, I replaced the lid and left the apartment with a great sense of satisfaction.

A few weeks later, my next challenge was a plugged-up garbage disposal. My previous experience in a kitchen and with plugged-up garbage disposals led me to believe I should arm myself with the 10 inch end of a broomstick that the owners had left for such occasions. Again, I had never been in this particular apartment. Mrs. K. was preparing a large family dinner for the upcoming Jewish holiday. She had peeled tons of potatoes and the peelings had successfully disabled the garbage disposal. Wonderful smells led me directly to the kitchen and I located the offending device. While digging through the peels, I suggested that the trash was really a better place to put them rather than the sink. I inserted my garbage unjamming tool into the drain and rocked the disposal unit gently back and forth until it loosened. I confidently, but sweetly, advised her that large amounts of any kind of peelings were really not good for a kitchen disposal. I could say this confidently as I had just been given this advice by a plumber after I had done the very same thing. She accepted my comments graciously and in turn told me about her family gathering and how her sons had been circumcised on the very same table that she would be setting. I had made another friend.

Chapter Seven

Kids, Toys and Challenges

Parenting is, without a doubt, one of the most rewarding, yet difficult and challenging responsibilities that a person can assume. It is also a responsibility for which we receive very little training. The tendency is to use the same parenting skills, or lack thereof, that were used by our own parents. I have managed to raise two sons of whom I am very proud. The two most important days in my life were the birth dates of my two sons. I wanted these two children and had no qualms about raising them as a blind mom. Being a good parent has nothing to do with a person's visual acuity. It has to do with wanting and loving your children. It has to do with having the confidence to know that for whatever problem arises there will be a solution.

I had no previous experience taking care of babies; but from the first diaper change and the first bath given I was confident I could do this. When my babies were sleeping, I frequently stood by the crib and listened to their breathing. That was my indication that all was well. When diapers were soggy or ear infections developed the cry was an obvious message that something needed to be done.

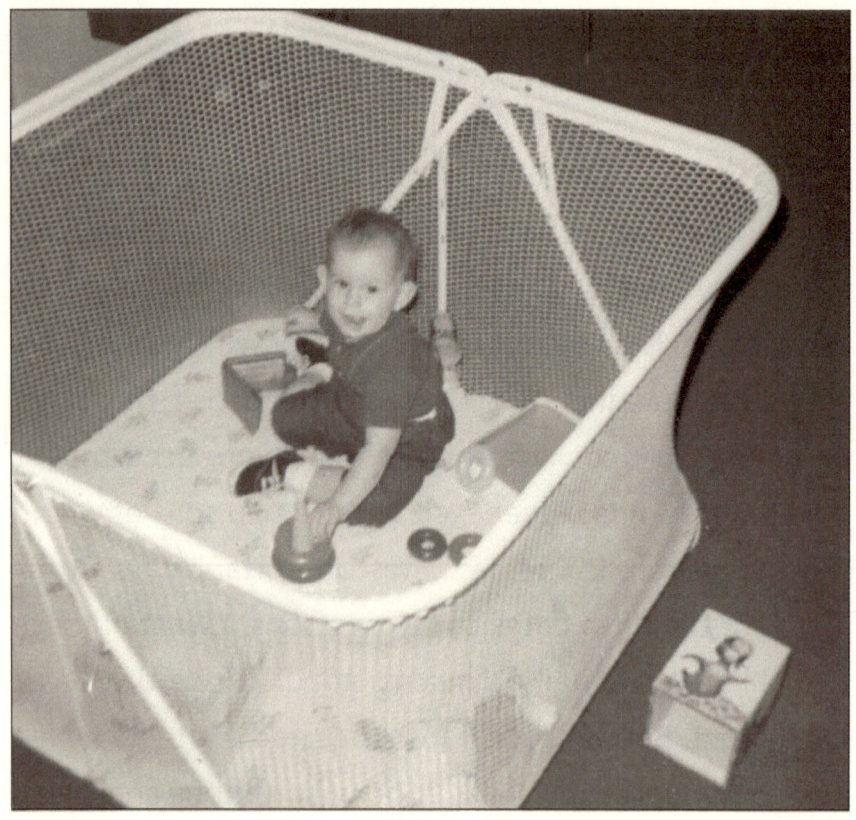

Kevin

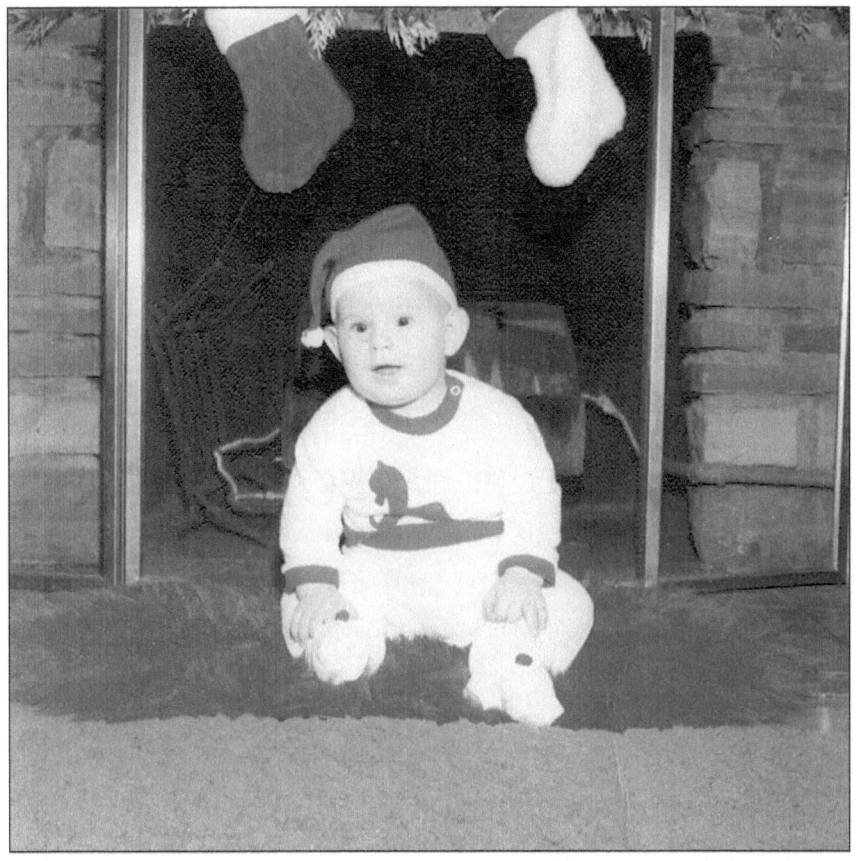

Jeff

As my babies learned to crawl and pull themselves up, I again depended upon my hearing. I must remind you once more that my hearing was no better than average; I simply learned to use it in a more efficient way. I completely child-proofed my house. I put all dangerous cleaners and household chemicals on high shelves far out of the reach of children. I never had to rush either of my boys to the hospital as a result of carelessness or improper care.

I have always been well organized and this became

a critical factor as a parent. Toys and games were always placed on appropriate shelves. There were, of course, times when toys would be strewn over the floor. I simply learned to sort of scoot my feet without destroying a special toy or stepping on a tiny finger.

The innocent and rather concrete thinking of a child is wonderful to observe. When Jeff was maybe three or four he had wanted to go outside and play. It had been raining and I told him that he couldn't go outside because of the rain and the ground was wet. "Can't you dry it"? he asked. For an instant I saw myself in the back yard with a huge bath towel drying off the grass. Another such conversation took place when my two boys and I were going somewhere with my mother. It was in the evening and Mom commented that the moon was full. Kevin asked her "Did it eat too much"?

When my boys became ready for Kindergarten, I walked them to school for the first several days. We were fortunate enough to live close to a neighborhood elementary school. In addition to teaching my boys the way to school I wanted to maintain a high profile and be a positive image for my kids. I suspected they would hear comments about their "blind mom." I became actively involved in PTA which I felt helped to create the image I desired. I just wanted to be a regular mom. I baked cookies for bake sales and worked at the school carnival. I served as PTA president.

I remember a conversation I had with Jeff, my older son, when he was in fifth grade. He told me that someone at school said, "I feel sorry for you because your mom is blind." When Jeff asked why, the boy responded, "Because you have to do all that cleaning and work at home." Jeff answered, "In the first place I don't know how to do all of that stuff and besides my mom does it all."

As they grew so did my challenges. It became important for me to know where they were as they grew old enough to leave the house. They learned this early and were usually pretty good about telling me where they were going and with whom. We lived in a fairly close-knit and safe neighborhood. If I needed to check up on one of them, I could usually count on a neighbor to track him down. As with all parents, child rearing is a most challenging proposition.

My boys learned early on that mom needed to look at things with her hands. They also learned that since they could not make direct eye contact with me, they needed to find other ways of getting my attention, and so they did. If I were in a conversation with someone, or speaking on the phone, they would tap me on the arm. If I ignored them, the tapping became faster and faster. I could determine the urgency of their concern by the intensity of their taps;

it worked. As they grew, so did the size of their toys. Often times as I entered the living room I would hear "Stop Mom! We are playing with our hot wheels." They would have successfully crisscrossed the entire room with tracks and didn't want all of their work wiped out. They loved playing out-of-doors and big wheels were their favorite mode of transportation for several years. The back yard and driveway became their well traveled road. During one of these play days they dug a rather sizable hole under the huge old fig tree. They enjoyed driving through the hole as part of their obstacle course. The day they decided to fill the hole with water from the garden hose was the beginning of a new challenge. Not only were their vehicles covered with mud but so were they. After such a day in the mud hole, I would peel off their clothes on the patio and rush them quickly into the bathtub.

When my boys were still quite young their father and I decided to go our separate ways. Relationships are a dynamic and ever-changing process. My husband was a good provider but after a few years something seemed to be lacking in our marriage. I did a great deal of soul-searching before this separation and divorce. Because of my divorced parents, I had promised myself I would never divorce, particularly if I had children. So much for promises. I was given total custody of Jeff and Kevin. Challenges increased but the three of us managed to persevere. The boys were each given tasks such as helping with dishes and taking out trash. Jeff had a paper route and Kevin began working in an Optometrist's office at the age of sixteen. He went on to become an optician. I did not want to stay at home and become a welfare mom, so I soon began looking for work. My first job was teaching Braille at a residential program for blind adults. Those times were tough but we all made it through. Money was always scarce but I felt good about working and providing for my children.

Schedules were tight. I took buses to work and the trip was an hour or more each way. Quite often I would prepare a meatloaf, or something, in the evening. I would tell Kevin what time to put it into the oven on the following day and this helped with dinner preparation. The crock pot became a wonderful friend. It was so good to step into my house and smell dinner all ready to go.

I held a BA in Sociology and had always wanted to work in the field of rehabilitation. That dream would take some time to be realized. My desire was to work in civil service in order to have the benefits for my sons and me. I got my foot into the door when I went to work for the California Department of Motor Vehicles. A likely job you say for a blind person? As you might suspect I was not hired to give drive tests. I worked in the information unit and answered vehicle related questions by phone. I used Braille cards to maintain the necessary information. It was a good job and it was civil service. After working for DMV for five years I applied for a counseling position with the Department of Rehabilitation and was hired as a counselor for blind and visually impaired clients.

Living with and caring for my sons has been a wonderful experience. I know it was tough on them growing up from ages six and nine without a dad. I am a firm believer in the fact that there is a reason for everything and that we have the opportunity to learn from every experience. If I had known then what I now know I am sure that I would have done some things differently. The good news is that my sons are grown and we have all moved ahead. Jeff is a computer technician and Kevin works in the television industry, and I am remarried, retired and happy.

CHAPTER EIGHT

My Empty Nest

As my two boys grew and matured, I began to dread the thought of them leaving home. It was inevitable, I knew, but I did not look forward to that eventuality.

Jeff, my older son, was the first to leave. He moved in with some friends who helped to share expenses. His work ethic was always good. He had a newspaper route when only ten or twelve years old. His customers rewarded him generously during the Christmas season. They appreciated the way he always placed the newspaper exactly where they wanted it. Jeff is now into computers and can run circles around me with his computer skills. If I run into a computer glitch, or the fax won't work, he's the one I call.

After Jeff left home, it seemed strange with only

Kevin and me. The two of us grew very close and shared a lot of household responsibilities. At an early age, he began baking cookies and cakes and has become a gourmet cook. We often shared in the preparation of meals.

Kevin was a fairly fussy eater, while his brother would eat just about anything. When I made stew, Kevin didn't want his meat touching his potatoes or any other vegetable. The other vegetables usually got left behind anyway. They both loved Jell-O, especially with sliced bananas. I made it fairly often. When you put a serving spoon into a freshly-made bowl of Jello and lift it out, it makes a sort of smacking noise. The boys loved that sound and called it Jello kisses. All I had to do was to take a bowl of Jell-O from the refrigerator, place it on the counter, and they would both come running, exclaiming, "I want to hear the Jell-O kisses!" I believe that there were some tough times for my boys growing up with a blind mom, but I also believe that this fact has made a positive difference in their lives. I couldn't be more pleased with my two sons, but I digress; back to the harsh realities of them leaving home.

Kevin became an optician and began saving money to move out on his own. That day finally came, and I was devastated. The two of us had grown very close. Now my family, living at home, was down to one. The big day came and Kevin moved into his upscale bachelor apartment. I gathered up some pots, pans and dishes, as I had done for Jeff. These times were so exciting for them, but inside mom there was a lot of sadness.

When I returned from work, turned the key in the lock, opened the door, and stepped into an empty house, I wondered how I would ever get through this transition. I knew I would, but how? I had been toying with the idea of returning to school to work on my Masters degree in Counseling and Psychology and thought this might be the time. Did I really want to go back to school in my 50's? I spoke to one of the counselors at a school where I was applying and she told me they had just graduated an eighty year-old woman with her Masters in Psychology. I took the plunge, applied, and was accepted to the graduate program.

My first semester was tough. I was still working full time and taking classes at night. I worked, went to class and studied. My social life disappeared, but I was enjoying the challenge. I began finding some perks to living alone. I could spread out my texts (which were on audio cassette), tape recorder and Braille notes all over the sofa or table and they were still in place when I returned home. My silent house soon became a haven for studying. There were other advantages I discovered. I could put food in the refrigerator, and it would be there when I returned. My two boys had a way of changing a well-stocked refrigerator into a vast wasteland. But even with these noted pluses, I frequently thought it would be nice to have a little more clutter in my life and my boys back home.

With the end of the first semester nearing, I was now looking at my first Christmas alone. I knew I would not be by myself on Christmas day, but what about all that baking, decorating and the other stuff that goes along with Christmas and kids? I debated whether or not to even get a Christmas tree. One day after work, Lee, a co-worker, surprised me and said he was taking me to pick out a tree. We found the right tree, brought it home, and he put it in the stand for me. He had time to put up the first string of lights before he had to leave. I thanked him and told him I could finish. I had always decorated the tree before the kids became old enough to really help. Kevin had taken on that task and, for the past several years, he had done the complete tree by himself.

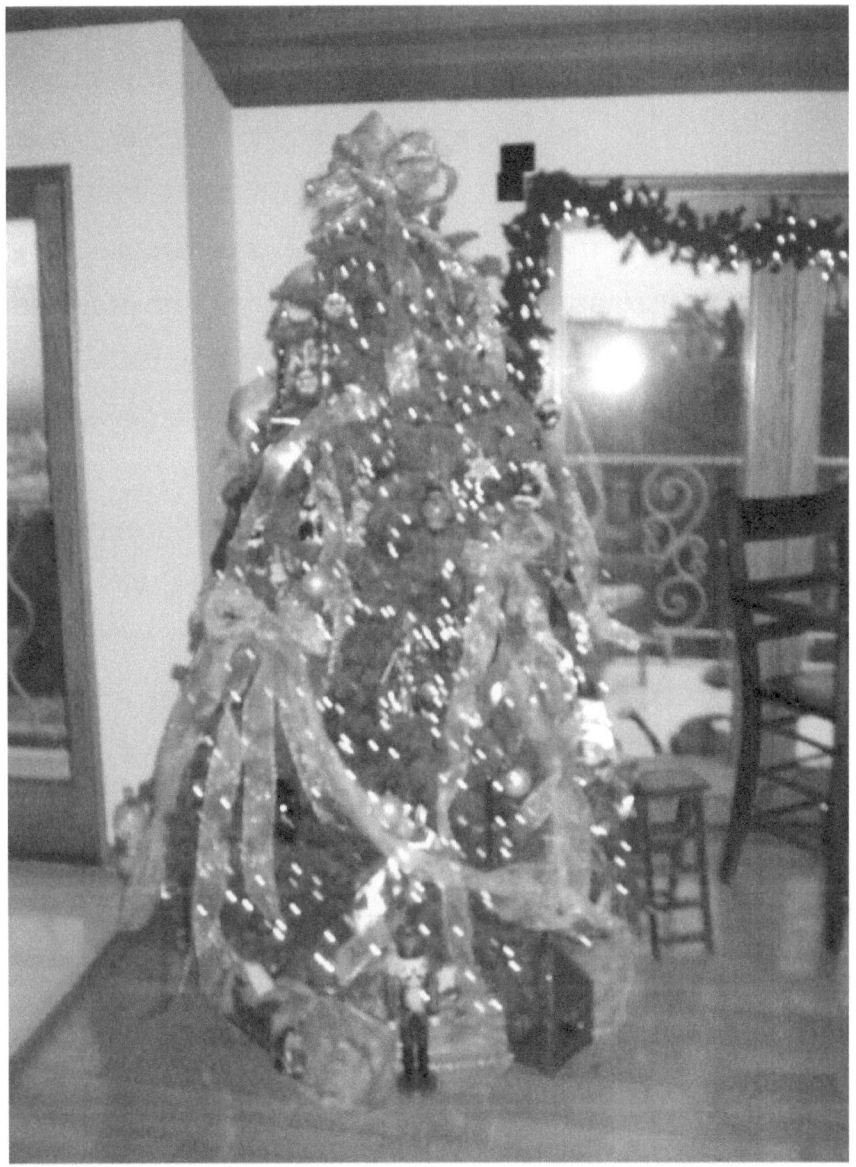

Kevin's Tree

I dragged out the boxes of brightly colored decorations. I sat on the floor among shiny balls, ornaments of all kinds (some made by my boys), and began to cry. How would I ever survive this Christmas?

Holidays, such as Christmas, Easter and Thanksgiving, were all celebrated with my family. My sister and I took turns putting together the Thanksgiving dinners. Christmas and Easter holidays sort of bounced around from my house to my sister's and my mother's. I can't remember exactly where I spent that first Christmas after my boys left, but I know it was with family.

I did survive, and I did complete my graduate courses and received my Masters degree. Sometimes, when we are staring at challenges, we have the tendency to run. I have learned that by meeting such challenges head on so much is to be gained. A problem is merely a way to get you to look at a situation differently. My philosophy of life is that for every problem there is a solution. The solution is not always readily recognizable, but it does exist.

My graduate courses got me back into reading, and I am always within reach of a good book. There is so much out there to be learned. I see myself as a student of life, and I hope never to stop learning. Along with that I have been given the gift of teaching. I find nothing more rewarding than to put my experiences as a blind woman to use. To make a positive difference in someone's life (particularly someone struggling with vision loss) is like the ultimate stroll on the cosmic beach of life. This is my purpose, this is my gift, and I give it away lovingly.

CHAPTER NINE

A Little Common Sense

There is a nearly universal belief system, or paradigm if you will, that says if someone is "different" that person is to be looked upon as inferior or is to be avoided completely. Television ads tell us how to dress, what breakfast cereal to eat and which toothpaste will make our smile whiter and brighter. And mostly we buy into this. There are, however, much less subtle, but just as effective ways of impacting people's belief systems. These subtle behavior patterns are often negative and harmful. The condescending way of speaking to an elderly woman or to someone in a wheelchair; speaking to the sighted companion rather than addressing the blind person who is making the transaction; or simply ignoring an individual with a disability are all examples of these subtle behavior patterns. These kinds of things occur all too frequently. I know, as I am blind and experience these incidents all too often. It is as if a person sees me and immediately begins to make assumptions. They assume (at least it seems that way from my experiences) that I must also be deaf as they often raise their voice. People also seem to assume that I may be mentally delayed and think I may not be able to make my own decisions or think for myself. They in their infinite wisdom want to do my thinking for me. Social conditioning is a powerful force and it is difficult to break through this force. For decades I have attempted to bring about awareness and to paint a more realistic view of vision loss and blindness. The writing of this book is another effort to continue my work on this daunting task.

I travel frequently with my husband Don (who also happens to be blind) and we are quite familiar with airline policies and procedures. In a recent trip, we checked in with the ticket agent and everything seemed to go smoothly. He asked if we needed assistance to get to the gate and we responded that we were familiar with the airport and could manage. I had written the flight information and seating assignments in Braille. We were assigned to row nine, seats E and F. We counted back to the ninth row and took our seats. Soon a woman was discussing with the flight attendant the fact that we were in her assigned seat.

Don pulled our tickets from his pocket and guess what? The ticket agent (well-meaning I'm sure) had moved us up to the third row and did not bother to inform us of this change. Apparently, he felt the third row would be more convenient for us regardless of our opinions. The incident became rather embarrassing as people around us probably jumped to the conclusion that since we were blind we could not possibly be expected to find our assigned seats. I can only suppose that the ticket agent felt that the third row would be more convenient for us but all he did was to create some confusion.

This kind of social unawareness has been passed down through generations. I understand that people are sometimes uncomfortable because of the lack of eye contact. We live in a visually oriented world—I get that. I also understand that there is a fear factor related to blindness. Surveys have shown that blindness is the most feared condition only after cancer and AIDS. When interacting with a blind person, some people are just out of their comfort zone but why is it that any common sense seems to take flight?

Another airline incident occurred when my friend Fred was on a recent cross-country flight. Fred, who happens to be blind (and also holds a Ph.D. in rehabilitation), takes frequent business-related trips. As he returned to his seat after visiting the lavatory, a flight attendant expressed her surprise at his ability to return to his assigned seat. It is very easy for a blind person to find his seat by touching and counting each row. As a matter of fact, it would be difficult for a blind person to get lost in a narrow airplane aisle.

Recently Don and I went to breakfast with some friends. The waitress began taking orders from my friends on the other side of the table and worked her way around to me. I gave the waitress my order with a fair amount of detail, but had apparently not covered one of the options. The waitress then addressed my friend (sitting across from me) and asked, "Does she want the full plate or just the half order"? I responded, "You might want to ask me." I was somewhat surprised at this particular assumption on the part of the waitress as we had been engaged in conversation about my order. Although I was quick to respond to the waitress, how do you suppose this made me feel in the pit of my stomach? I am being treated, in front of my friends, as an inferior human being. If these kinds of incidents occurred infrequently there would be no concern.

You may be thinking that too much is being made of these incidents. Put yourself in my position and see how this plays out. As an adult, is it not demeaning and patronizing to be completely ignored by the person with whom you are speaking? I have been in this position all too often. I have been in meetings with professionals when agendas or other paperwork is being passed around. Such paperwork has often been passed over my head, or behind my back. As an educated blind woman, I obviously must have a way of accessing printed materials. At such times, however, these strange assumptions seem to kick in and my presence is ignored until I object. I have had blind friends say to me when these kinds of incidents occur that it makes them feel like a "nothing."

Some weeks later Don and I were again eating breakfast out with some friends. This was a different location and a different waitress. As she was ready to take my order, she placed her hand on my shoulder and asked, "And what would you like"? This waitress got it. No false assumptions on her part. I will never know the thought process of the first waitress but it seems to be another of those all too frequent instances of the lack of common sense. My friends were as astonished and amazed as I. Contrast that conversation with that of the second waitress and see what difference a tiny, but thoughtful, gesture can make.

As I describe these incidents I suspect most readers will get it. I realize that part of the problem is the lack of contact that society has with blind and visually impaired people. The blind population is a minority group, in every sense of the word, experiencing the same kinds of discrimination that other minorities experience. However, the attitudes directed towards blind people are generally based on pity and fear (fear of vision loss) as opposed to distrust or dislike. The root of the problem with any of these stereotypes is ignorance and lack of understanding. My lifelong goal has been to bring some understanding to the general public and to convince people that it just takes a little common sense.

CHAPTER TEN

My Career as a Photographer

As a child, like most children, I was very curious and very observant. I enjoyed looking at cloud formations and loved getting a glimpse of a rainbow. One of my fondest memories is waking up in my grandmother's house and looking out the window after a new snow had fallen. The white blanket gently covered everything in sight. It draped the otherwise bare limbs of the trees. The snow was so beautiful before it was walked upon and before it began to melt.

Other fond memories include the Christmas that I received my shiny new bicycle. I enjoyed bike riding, swimming, and roller skating. I watched with interest as my grandmother made biscuits or bread. She would take a handful of this and a pinch of that. At about the age of nine, I was successfully throwing together biscuits just as she did. I read and traded comic books with my cousin. I was an avid reader and read just about any book I could get my hands on. I was not good at drawing or painting. I remember showing my mother (who's nature tended to be rather critical) a picture of the little red car I had drawn. I thought it was a fine car. Did it really matter if the wheels were not exactly rounding? One thing is for sure that the world did not lose an artist, in the traditional sense of the word, when I lost my sight at the age of eleven. It was much later in my life when I recognized my true artistic abilities.

Another of my childhood interests was photography. I loved the idea of pointing that little box at something, snapping the picture, getting the film processed, and then seeing a reproduction of the scene. This career, however, was short-lived because of the injury that caused my blindness. The camera was put away along with my bike and roller skates. As I matured and adjusted to my blindness, I still loved having pictures around. I like having people describe a picture to me so that I can paint an image in my mind.

After marrying and having two sons, pictures became an even more important part of my life. My husband or some family member was always taking pictures and would then arrange them in an album for safekeeping. I must have passed this interest on, as both of my sons enjoy photography. Photos of family members are placed throughout my home. I have pictures of palm trees and bubbling waterfalls that were taken on a vacation trip to Hawaii. In an album, somewhere, there is a picture of my younger son, Kevin, sitting in his highchair, leaning over and dumping a spoonful of oatmeal onto his foot. In that same album are pictures of his brother Jeff, in his Cub Scout uniform. Photographs are a wonderful tool for preserving history.

When my boys were fairly young, their father and I agreed to go our separate ways. I was given full custody of my children. Much later after both boys were grown and on their own, I remarried. I moved from California to New Mexico for a short time where, Don, my new husband lived. I immediately fell in love with the Native American culture and began collecting brightly colored pictures, pottery, and Indian rugs to decorate our home. I soon became quite comfortable in our 100 year-old adobe house.

Don had lost most of his sight at the age of 50 due to macular degeneration[8]. He has some functional vision in one eye but is technically legally blind. He could no longer drive and was forced out of his long career in industrial construction. We lived in New Mexico for about a year and then returned to California. After retiring, we moved back to New Mexico, where we currently reside.

During my very first winter in New Mexico, it snowed on October 31st. I had not been in snow since I was a kid in Missouri, where I grew up. I was so excited that I dragged Don outside into the white fluffy stuff. We made snowballs and threw them at each other. He stopped and ran into the house and grabbed the camera. He took several shots of me enjoying the new snow. I sort of sadly lamented that I could not take his picture. Don said that I could. I argued that I could not. He handed me the camera. I remembered how to hold it and to focus. Don said that he would talk to me so that I would know where to aim. He did, and I did. It was at that moment that my career as a photographer was reclaimed.

This entire episode in my life was another wonderful learning experience. Here I was quite adjusted to my vision loss, but still insisting there were things I could not do. I have spent most of my life working with other blind people, convincing them to concentrate on the things they could do and not to focus on the things they could not do. There I was telling myself that I could not ... Since that day I have taken hundreds of pictures and most of them are right on target. Sometimes I aim a little high or to the side, but much of the time I am right on. When there is no one else around to do so, I take the pictures.

Don loves to garden and spends many hours working in the yard. In our back yard a tree had grown up much too close to a block wall. Don felt that the tree needed to come down and gathered his saw and a ladder. The tallest limbs were actually growing into the telephone and power lines and he had to saw and carefully maneuver the limbs through the lines. After his first few cuts with the saw, I decided to take pictures of this process. While he was on the ladder, I had him talk to me, and I pointed the camera in the direction of his voice and the sound of the saw. I suddenly began to laugh. Don wanted to know what was so funny. I explained, "No one will believe this. Here is a blind guy on a ladder cutting down a tree and his blind wife is in the yard taking pictures." The resulting photos showed the process from start to finish. I over-shot on only one picture as I had aimed too high.

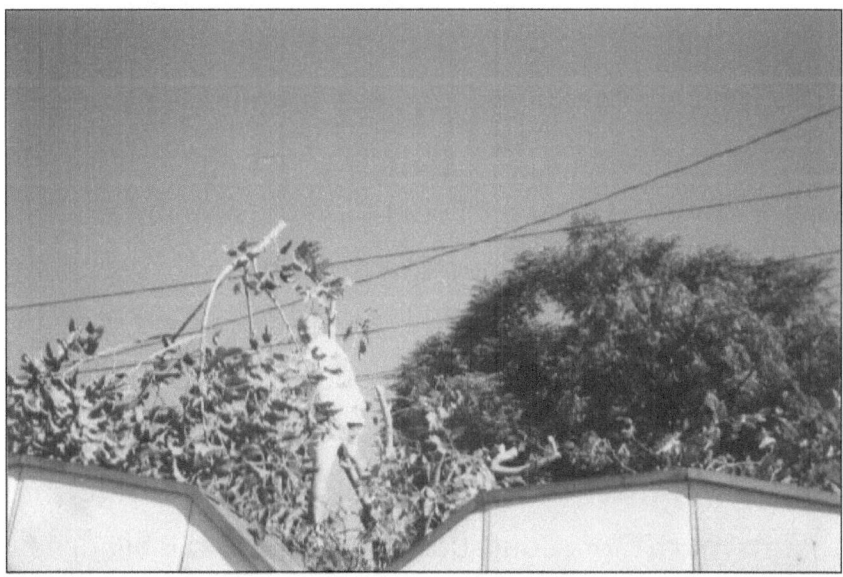

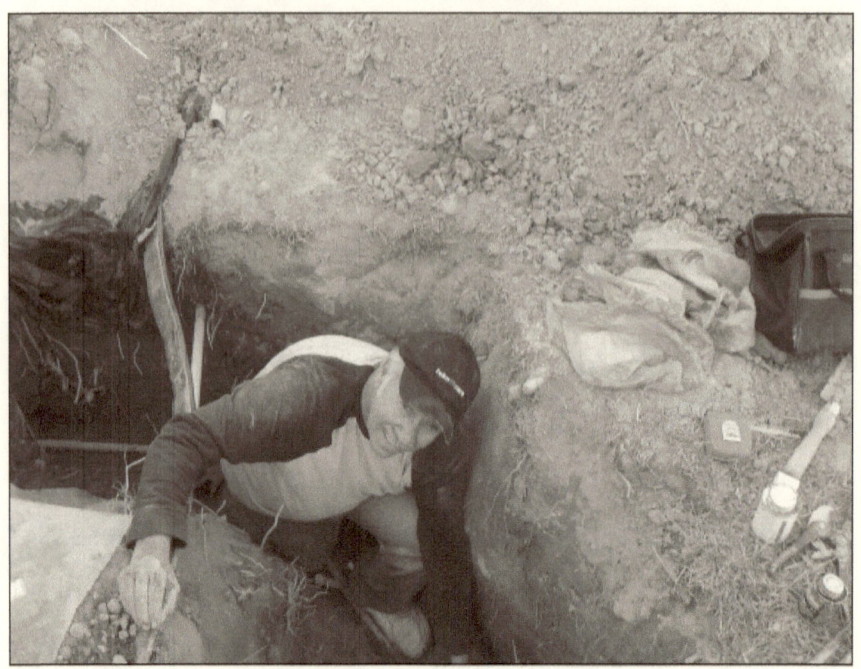

Photos by Nancy

These skills and abilities did not come to me overnight. As a newly blinded child, I was lost and unsure of myself. As an adult, I am confident, competent, and still learning. A great deal of encouragement was given to me along the way. I found the National Federation of the Blind while in college. Wonderful friends and mentors, who happened to be blind, encouraged and inspired me. I owe much of my philosophy of life to these supportive blind sisters and brothers.

As I reflect back on this experience I realize that there is much more education to be done about blindness. Unfortunately, society still holds many incorrect beliefs about blind or visually impaired people. We will have made progress when the tree trimming, photo taking experience is no longer seen as absurd.

CHAPTER ELEVEN

Release the Artist Within

Open your mind. Tap into your creativity. All of us have been given unique talents and gifts. Sometimes these gifts lay buried under what feels like a ton of responsibility or simply have never been acknowledged. If you enjoy doodling or sketching, perhaps you have the soul of an artist. Tap into this gift on a daily basis. If it feels right, keep watching your gift blossom and grow.

Talents and gifts come in assorted packages. It isn't necessary to be able to draw or paint or write to be considered an artist. As I mentioned earlier, I was sure the world had not lost an artist when I lost my sight. I am, however, able to express my creativity in many ways. Obviously, I enjoy writing and am able to do so, on a computer equipped with synthetic speech. While in school and college I wrote papers first on a manual typewriter (my very own Underwood portable to be specific). Later, I used an electric one with correction tape. I thought that the ability to correct without using "white out" was the greatest gift since sliced bread.

This discussion reminds me of an incident that took place while I was attending the school for the blind. In a ninth grade English class we spent several months working on essays. The teacher required us to turn in an essay every week. I loved writing and always managed to complete my assignment quickly. Julie, a good friend of mine, did not like writing and often asked me to help with her essays. She would give me a topic and then I would write the entire essay for her. I would try to do this from her perspective and as far as we know, our English teacher never suspected the conspiracy.

But to get on with my creativity, I love home decorating. Living in the American southwest, I enjoy displaying colorful Indian rugs which hang on the walls. Pottery and Indian artifacts are scattered throughout my home. It gives me a great deal of satisfaction to add Native American items or to arrange and rearrange existing pictures or collectibles. Entertaining, cooking, and particularly baking, are sources of pleasure to me. I am happy if I have a birthday party or a Thanksgiving dinner to plan. I love setting a pretty table with linens and china.

Since my move to Albuquerque, however, I have exchanged my pastel-colored China for the vivid and brightly colored Fiesta ware. I enjoy working out a menu and preparing for the big event. Give me a function to organize and I will tap into every ounce of creativity I possess.

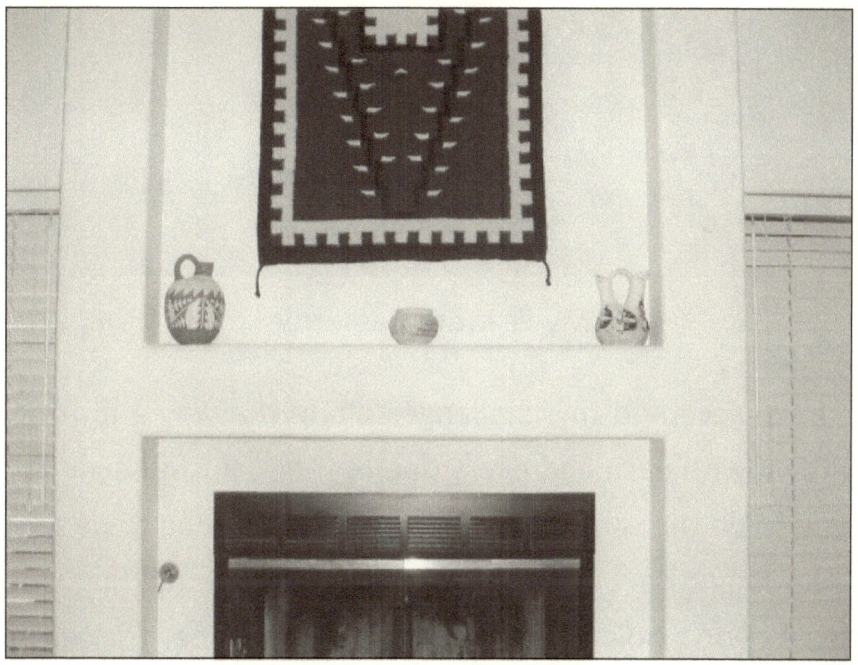

A Touch of Southwest Decor

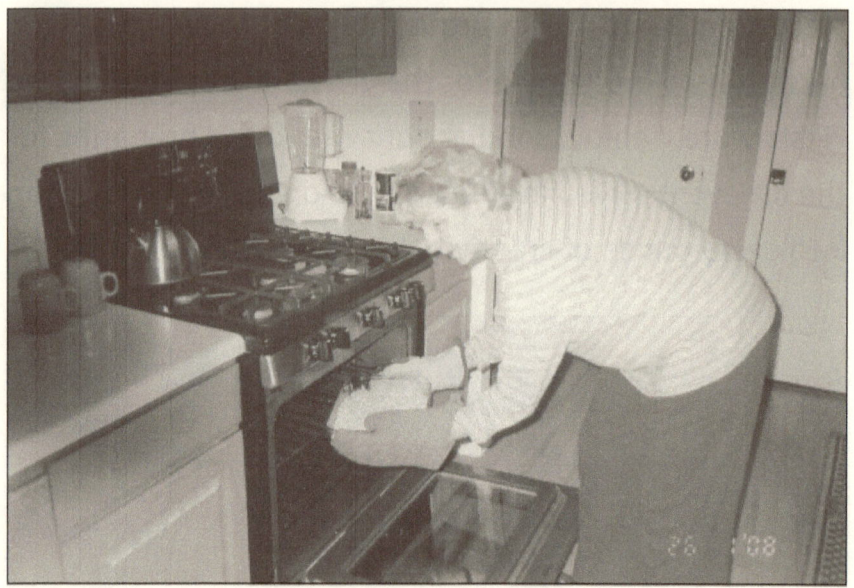

My Favorite Casserole

I have accepted my challenges along the way and have grown with each and every one of them. It is possible for you to do the same and I am not only speaking to people who might have a disability, but to anyone reading this book. Don't hold back. Live at risk. Remember that each small success is a stepping stone to a larger success. Reach for the stars for they are within your grasp.

CHAPTER TWELVE

The Dark Side of Disability

Because of my own personal experiences and my professional work with blind and other disabled people, I believe there are issues of great importance which are frequently avoided. It is not uncommon for people in the disabled population to be sexually, physically, mentally, and financially abused. All too often this population is dependent upon others, and herein lays the problem. Generally speaking, young children totally trust older adults. Unfortunately, this should not always be the case. It is up to parents to carefully secure the confidence of their own children and to take steps to ensure their safety. Communication is the key. This is even more important for a child with a disability than it is for a non-disabled child.

As a blind teenager living at home I was sexually

abused by my alcoholic stepfather. This man was physically abusive to my mother but she was apparently unable to find the strength or support needed to deal with the circumstances. I was convinced that if I had gone to the authorities to report either situation that he would have killed me. This may or may not have been the truth but this totally abusive man had me convinced.

Because of these experiences I researched the subject while in my graduate program. There were not a lot of studies, at least at that time, on this issue as it related to the blind population. There was, however, a fair amount of information about such abuse in the deaf community. If a deaf child has no verbal skills, how can he ask for help?

All of this is, indeed, the bad news. The good news is that as a counselor working with young blind women I could quickly identify the evidence of abuse. My own personal experience with abuse allowed me to recognize symptoms as they manifested themselves in my clients. Abuse happens all too often. Unsuspected family members or caretakers are frequently the violators. I will share just two specific tragic incidents to make my point; both of these young ladies were totally blind. The first young lady, approximately nineteen years of age, was extremely shy and timid. As we established a positive rapport she shared with me the facts of her living arrangements. She had been sent to live with an aunt and uncle who required her to do all the cooking and cleaning for the household. In addition to that she was required to have frequent sex with her uncle. Other disturbing factors became evident. She never had proper clothing and even in cold weather she arrived without a jacket or warm clothes.

The second situation that I clearly remember revolved around an 18 year-old high school student living with her biological family. She too impressed me as someone living in an abusive situation. This student was made to do the cooking, cleaning and caring for her younger siblings but was never given any of her supplemental security income. Sexual abuse was also suspected. A concerned school teacher had gained her confidence and the girl had told her that she had shared this information with me. The teacher contacted me and together we worked out a plan to relocate her into a safe residential situation.

I was also able to relocate the first young woman. As determined as she was to leave her abusive situation, she still felt a strong obligation to this aunt and uncle and at the last minute I feared that her move would not happen. It did happen and as far as I know both of these young women are out of their abusive relationships. Hopefully they have managed to find additional support systems.

Victims of abuse often have difficulty severing

relationships with the aggressor. This fact is evident with all victims, not just those who may be disabled, particularly when it comes time to press charges against the perpetrator. In the two cases described above, as well as in my own case, the victims tended to search for the good side of the abuser. Support groups, such as Adults Molested as Children, are helpful but effects of abuse leave lasting emotional scars. This kind of abuse is not left behind easily. Such abuse should never happen to anyone but it all too often happens to those of us who are least able to defend ourselves. My own life has been permanently scarred even after hours of painful, although liberating, therapy and work in support groups.

If any person reading this book has the slightest indication that there might be an abusive situation involving a child, a friend, or a family member please contact the proper authorities. A child or young adult with a disability has much to learn in life. Don't allow the possibility of an abusive situation to be one of these lessons.

CHAPTER THIRTEEN

The Portrait

My injury, and resulting vision loss, was a tragedy not just to me but also to my mother. As I reflect back on those years during which I adjusted to my blindness, one thing becomes painfully clear. My mother did not. She was a woman who thrived on perfection. Her handwriting was beautiful. Her dress was immaculate. She demanded absolute obedience from her two children by the use of a furrowed-brow, cocked-jawed, stern expression that my sister and I refer to as "the look."

As a result of the desire to please our mother, my sister and I both have good taste in clothing and like to always appear well dressed. I was tall and lanky and if my mother spotted even a hint of a slouch she would pull my shoulders back and tell me to stand up straight. The unfortunate thing is that she was never good at verbal communication. Even after I could no longer see her I was aware of "the look." Because of her inability to communicate verbally with me, I never quite knew what to expect from her. Since my vision loss, I don't ever remember her using the word "blind." I am sure that this was because of her inability to deal with reality. She needed perfection and now one of her daughters was no longer perfect in her eyes. I am certain that she was in pain as she saw me struggle with my blindness. She just did not know how to handle the circumstances and apparently there was not a lot of support for her. Much of her childhood and youth are a mystery and will remain as such. We suspect that her childhood was not a happy one and that she built up some defenses which remained with her throughout her 96 years of life. Mom generally appeared to be happy as she had a wonderful sense of humor. She worked in the insurance field into her 70's. Mom made many friends in the work-place and maintained some of these friendships until the time of her death.

As long as most family members can recall, there have been two eleven by fourteen portraits of my sister and me displayed in Mother's living room. The best guess is that Jan was about seven years old in her portrait, which would have made me around thirteen or fourteen years old. I clearly remember a discussion between my mother and the photographer about my obviously injured eye. There was some discussion that the photographer might be able to touch it up, but in the end, the decision was made to take a profile, thus ensuring a "perfect" portrait. As a result of this photography session I have always disliked this particular picture and its constant reminder of my mother's inability to accept my blindness.

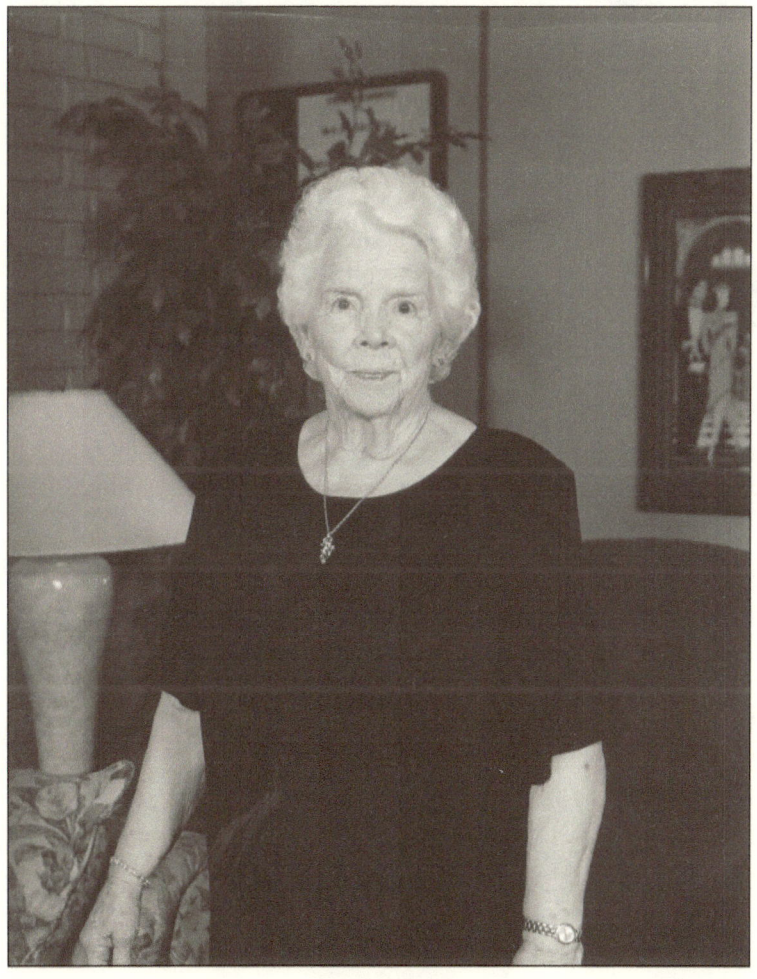

Mother

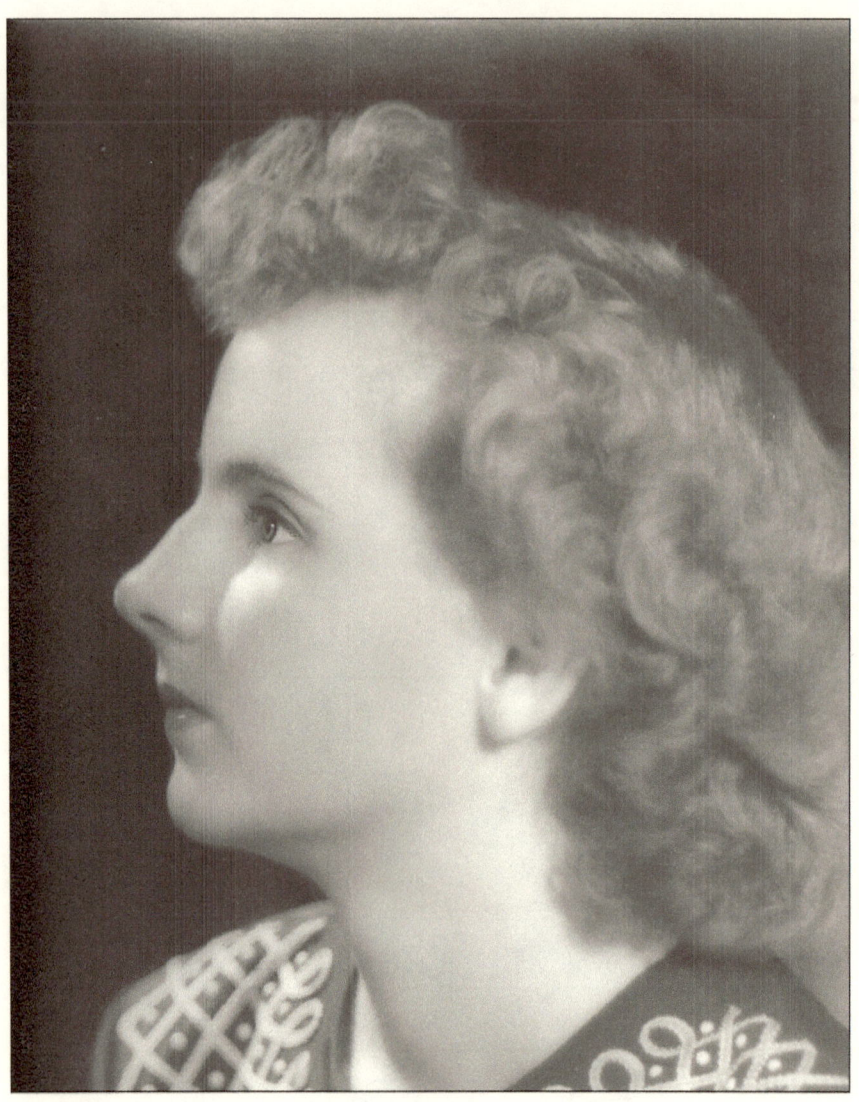

Nancy

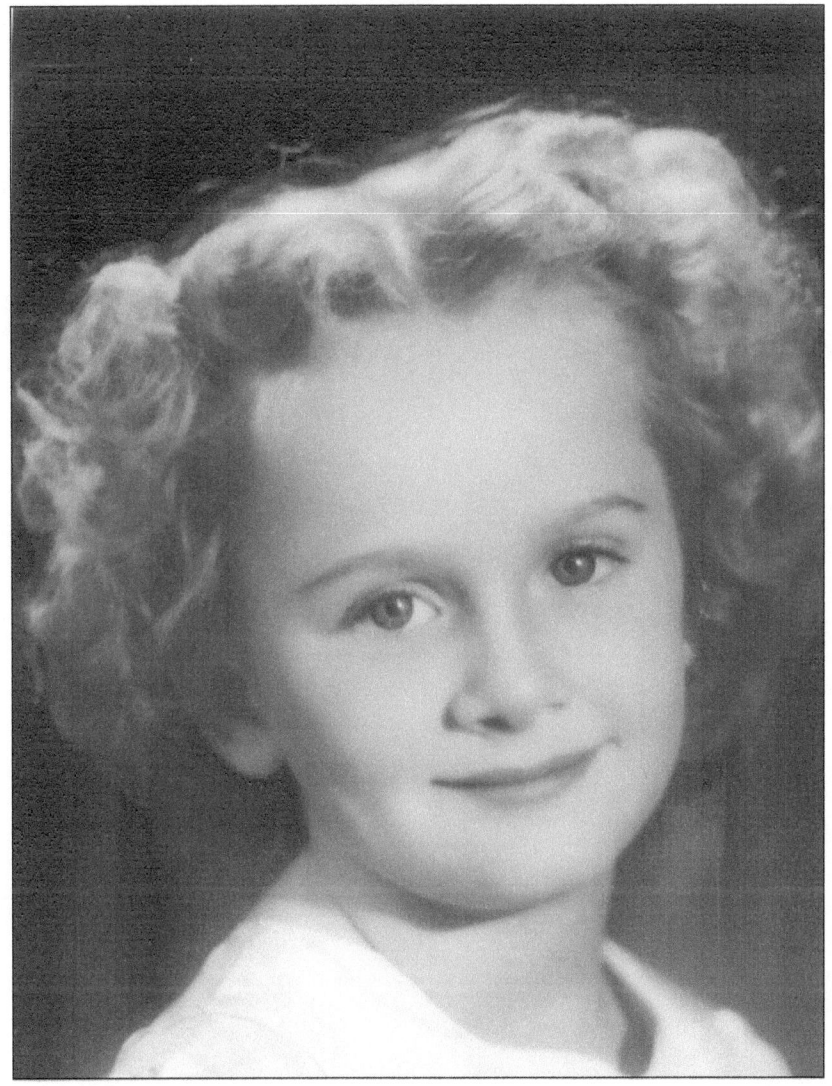

Janice

Now fast-forward some forty years and the introduction of Don into my family. Although legally blind, he is able to see this picture and he has always loved it. After my mother's death, Jan took her picture home. Don insisted on bringing mine to our new Albuquerque home. He reframed it and it now hangs on our living room wall after some objection from me. I had never shared the conversation at the photography session with anyone. But now that I have, I suppose I am okay with it hanging in plain view and with the rather sad history which lies behind it.

CHAPTER FOURTEEN

Mirror, Mirror on the Wall

The art of dressing, coordinating, and staying in fashion can sometimes be a little challenging without the use of a mirror. My Mother blessed me with the desire to look good and always fashionable. Remember, my philosophy of life is that for every problem there is a solution. Sometimes it takes a little time, work, and effort to find that solution but trust me it is always there.

My sister, Janice, has always been part of my solution. Although there is a seven year difference in our ages, we are very close. She is not only my sister—she is my best friend. We both like to shop and she has a good eye for colors. Sometimes I would even call her and ask, "What length of skirt is being shown? Or "What colors are in right now?" I have good visual recall of colors and have a pretty good idea of what goes with what. If I really need to match colors in a skirt and blouse, for example, I like to go shopping with Jan or with one of my friends whose judgment I trust.

I do recall one shopping trip with Don, (who by the way is a great shopper) when I found a great blazer on a sales rack. Don, because of his limited vision, is not so good with colors. There were two women shoppers within ear shot. I held up the jacket in question and asked the ladies their opinion of the color. It was a shade of blue and there are tons of shades of blue. They both eagerly described the color and even began to say what other colors would work with the blazer. I thanked them for their assistance. They both seemed to delight in giving their opinion and it was helpful to me. I have had other similar situations. If you give an individual the opportunity to help, that individual usually comes through and feels good about doing so.

I am often asked how I am able to select my clothes. I generally respond by saying something like this. If you go into your closet with the lights turned out and examine your clothes you will be surprised how many things you are able to identify by touch. There are so many different fabrics and styles. I do try not to buy two articles of clothing that are identical except for the color. Braille tags can be slipped into a blazer pocket or placed over the hanger to identify a particular outfit.

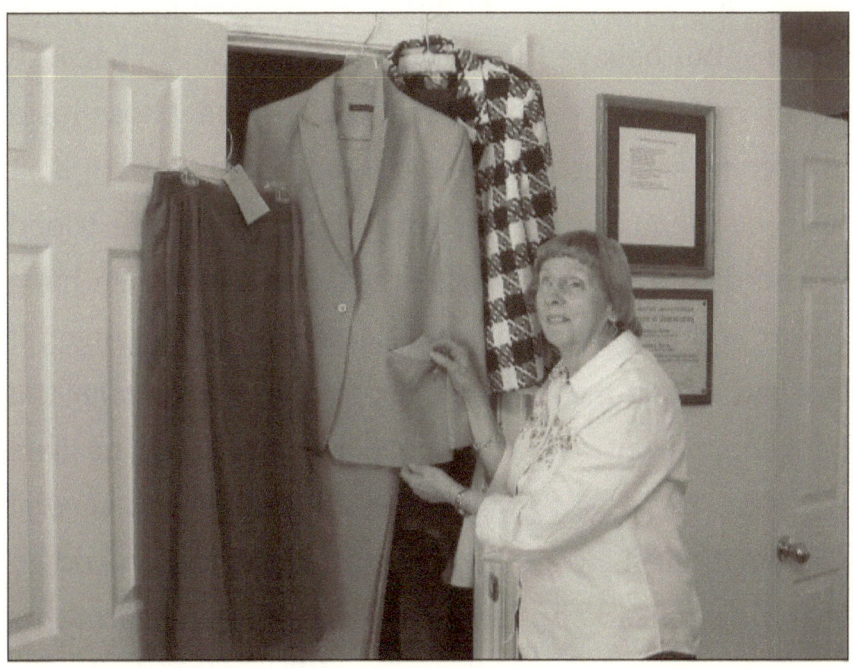

Braille Tags in a Pocket or on a Hanger Help to Coordinate my Wardrobe

Hair and makeup are simply a matter of a lot of practice. Of course, there are changing trends in these areas. It is again important to ask a friend or relative about these fashion changes. For some time now, I have purchased my makeup from the same individual and have grown to trust the opinion of this sales person.

I have facilitated numerous groups of women who are experiencing vision loss. Wardrobe management is always an important issue. One woman who had previously worked at a boutique on Rodeo Drive in Beverly Hills was very depressed. She lamented that she used to wear beautiful clothes with all kinds of accessories, such as scarves, but believed she could no longer do so because of her vision loss. I asked if she had a friend whose taste in clothing she trusted. She did. I suggested that the next time her friend came to her house she could ask the friend to coordinate some of her clothes. She might then hang a skirt and accompanying blouse on the same hanger. If she had a scarf that worked, it could be draped over the hanger and even include a lapel pin if so desired. She liked the idea. This works for me and if I do this with several combinations, I always have something to put on and go if an unexpected shopping trip or evening out presents itself. Remember, my philosophy of life is that for every problem there is a solution.

CHAPTER FIFTEEN

Dancing in Dallas

As I was completing my Masters in Counseling and Psychology, I was not sure of my next vocational objective. I just knew that I loved the subject matter that I was studying and felt that it would be useful in my future. I had taken an early retirement from the Department of Rehabilitation in order to complete my last semester. I found a part-time job which helped with finances.

As I mentioned earlier, I had been very involved in the National Federation of the Blind. I made arrangements to attend a national conference in Dallas, Texas and roomed with Pat, a long-time friend from California. Christine, another friend from California, now living in New Mexico, introduced me to Don. He seemed warm, polite and had a wonderful sense of humor. We kept meeting in various convention sessions and after-hour social gatherings. One of these chance meetings was at a Texas style barbecue. There was plenty of beer and food and a live western band. The dancing area was an outdoor grassy park. Don asked me to dance and before we knew it the evening was gone. The next day, which was the final day of the conference, we exchanged phone numbers and that was the beginning of a long-distance telephone romance. Don was from New Mexico; I was from California but fate put us together in Dallas, Texas. There was something magical about this relationship. He was warm and tender yet strong and rugged. I was captivated by his total attention to me. We were in our 50's and seemed to be quickly falling in love. Don and I were at the right place in our lives to make this wonderful gift work.

At the time of our meeting, neither of us even considered the possibility of finding a new soul mate. Don had worked in industrial construction most of his life and had been forced into retirement at the age of fifty because of his partial vision loss due to macular degeneration. He had been married and had a grown son and daughter. After his vision loss and forced retirement, his wife of twenty-eight years left. In addition to dealing with his vision loss, he had lost trust in women—until we met.

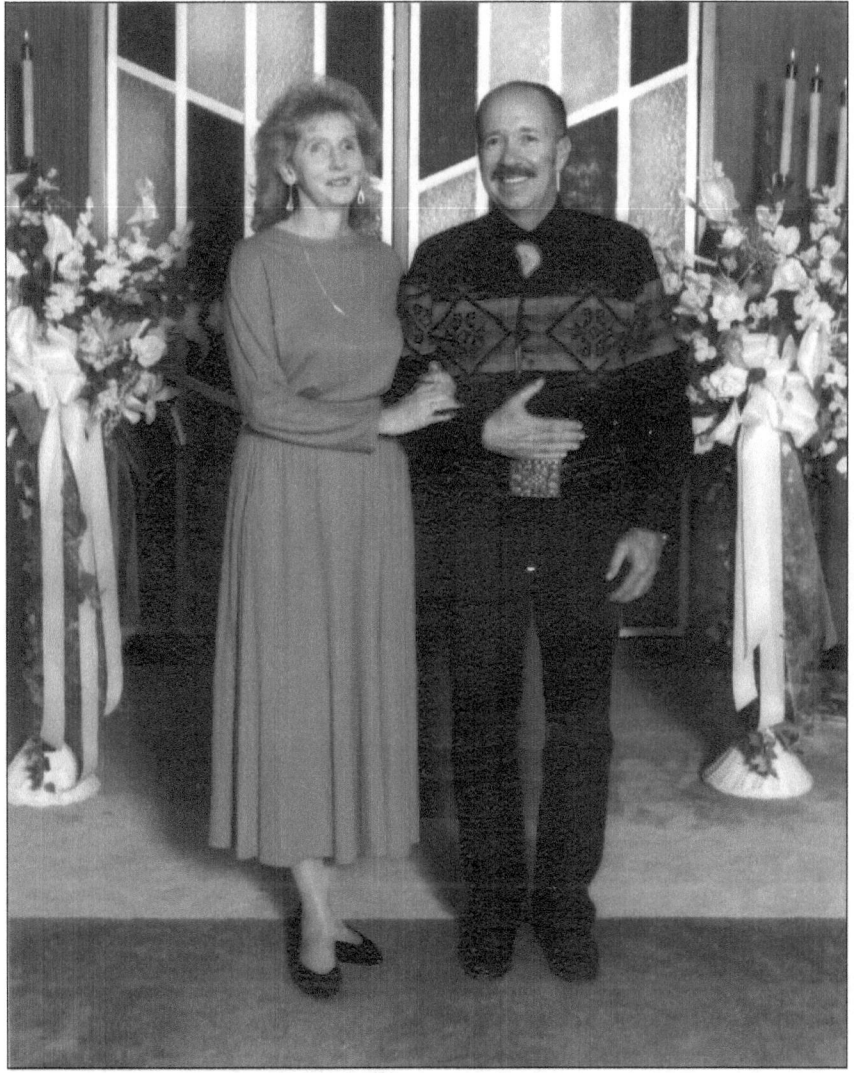

Married in Reno

Our first meeting was in July of 1993 and in October of that same year we were married. I moved to New Mexico and for a short time worked for the New Mexico Commission for the Blind as a counselor. We then moved to California where I still owned property and had family and many other connections. Don adjusted to life in Southern California quickly with one exception. That one exception was the lack of hot green chiles. There is a big difference between California style Mexican food and the Southwest cuisine found in New Mexico. The Southwest blends Spanish, Indian and Anglo recipes together to create spicy and colorful dishes. When dining out the waiter will ask "red or green." This refers to the red or green chiles that dominate New Mexico flavors. These chiles are grown only in New Mexico and are nowhere to be found in California. I would shudder when dining out and Don would order huevos rancheros or some other favorite dish. I found myself telling him to remember he was in California and not to expect the huevos, or whatever, to which he was accustomed.

Don is a wonderful gardener and finally resorted to growing the spicy chiles that he missed. He soon learned why they were not readily found in California. There is much too much humidity for these peppers to grow. It takes a hot and dry climate. The chile farmers in New Mexico grow the hottest peppers with the least amount of water. Don is not one to give up. The problem was solved by bringing back a suitcase full of frozen green chile each time we went to New Mexico.

Since the chile crisis was somewhat resolved, he turned his energy to creating a beautiful lawn bordered with flowers and many colorful roses. He had never been able to grow roses like that in New Mexico. He also had a vegetable garden in the back yard and was amazed at the size of the tomatoes he could grow. At the end of the season we were giving away bags of tomatoes to our neighbors. All of this because I went dancing in Dallas.

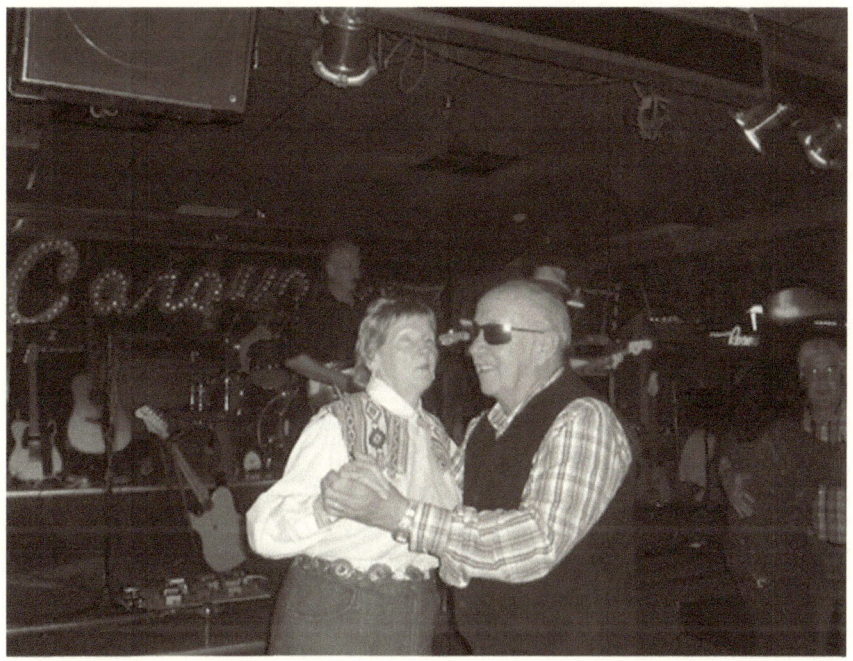

Dancing to Live Music in our Favorite Club

CHAPTER SIXTEEN

What Happened to Braille?

While living in California, Don and I were very involved in the NFB. I had served on the Board of Directors for many years and was elected state president in the fall of 2000. I served a six-year term. Don became the legislative representative for this organization and established a close rapport with the state legislature. His legislative career was outstanding with the passage of many laws which would have a positive impact on the lives of blind Californians. The high point in my last year as NFB of California president and Don's last year as the legislative advocate, was the passage of legislation which mandates Braille math and reading standards for blind students. These standards are equivalent to those mandated for sighted children in public schools. At the time of this writing, California is the only state which has such legislation. For a number of reasons, which include a teacher shortage and reluctance on the part of some parents to have their child learn Braille, only about ten percent of blind students are being taught Braille. The majority of legislators, along with the general public, had no idea that this was the case. It was simply believed that if a child was blind that child was being taught to read and write Braille.

With the over-crowding of residential schools and the resulting main-streaming of blind kids, the quality of education for blind students has plummeted. An itinerant teacher might work with a blind kid once or twice a week which is totally unacceptable. Sighted students are immersed in a print rich environment and reading generally comes easily. With the lack of instruction in the reading and writing of Braille, the prospects for success become quite diminished. Literacy is a strong predictor of success. Blind and visually impaired students were being deprived of this civil right.

During the process of lobbying for this legislation, many itinerant teachers who were not proficient in Braille became intimidated and also became opponents of the passage of this legislation. It was a long uphill battle to realize a successful conclusion. A total of seven years was devoted to this effort. The first bill, although passing through the California legislature, was vetoed by the

Governor. We knew our efforts were important and we did not go away until we had a successful bill passed and signed by Governor Schwarzenegger (AB2326).[9]

After these challenging and valuable successes, we were ready to again retire and relocate. I had made many trips to New Mexico with Don as he still had family there. We began to seriously consider moving to Albuquerque. This whole process from the sale of the California home to the purchase of our Albuquerque home went smoothly. It was hard for me to leave family and friends in California but we were accustomed to travel. We continue to financially support airline carriers between New Mexico and California.

Don is an out-of-doors kind of guy and loves his garden and can now grow green chile (hot ones). I enjoy shopping and decorating my new home. We both still love to go dancing and do so fairly often. I have more time to tap into my creativity through frequently entertaining my new-found friends and in my writing. We both continue to volunteer our services for the NFB but on a less regular basis.

CHAPTER SEVENTEEN

Cruisin' the Caribbean

Traveling to new places and exploring new environments have always been favorite activities of mine. I have been asked more than once how I am able to enjoy traveling. The assumption is, I suppose, that a person could not enjoy a trip without experiencing it visually. My response generally goes something like this: "I guess I could stay at home and just hear about the trips that others take but I choose not to do that." Trains, buses, planes, and ships-I have experienced them all, but my preference is sailing the seas. Whether it is a short trip from Long Beach to Catalina Island or a luxury cruise through the Caribbean, the ocean is my favorite place to vacation. I love the smell of the salt air and hearing waves break against the shore.

Don and I took our first cruise shortly after we

were married. That cruise around the Hawaiian Islands was all it took; we were hooked. We have since taken five more cruises. One of our recent trips was a seven-day cruise through the western Caribbean. We sailed from Ft. Lauderdale on a Sunday at 5 pm. About an hour or so into the trip we ran into a rather fierce storm. The huge Holland America ship bounced like a toy in the twenty-five foot waves. The ship pitched and rolled all that night and into the next day. It was the first time I had experienced an elevator moving from side to side as well as up and down at the same time. Ugh!

Our first island stop was to be Half Moon Cay; however, the waves were still so high we could not anchor and get into the tenders that would take us from the ship to the island. That evening the apologetic captain told us that he was sailing the ship into the leeward side of another island where he would drop anchor and we could all, including the captain, get a good night's sleep. The next morning the seas were calm and we set sail for Jamaica, which was still a day away. By the time we reached Ocho Rios, we had been on the ship for three nights and two full days. There were always shipboard activities, but an epidemic of cabin fever was evident as passengers poured off the ship for sightseeing or shopping trips.

The ship's theatre with Broadway-type musicals was always a pleasurable evening event. During the storm however, the show was cancelled because it was too dangerous for the singers and dancers to be on the stage. There were bingo games and a casino for the gamblers and shuffleboard was available on one of the decks. I always enjoyed the informative talks which gave information and points of interest about the next port. An on-ship store provided passengers with souvenirs and other necessities of life.

The next day our ship anchored at the Grand Cayman Islands. Tortuga rum and rum cakes are the sought-after items in Georgetown. I learned that the word Tortuga in Spanish means turtle. Christopher Columbus discovered these islands in 1503 and named them Las Tortugas because of the numerous turtles he observed. The name was later changed to Grand Cayman. The final stop before sailing back to Ft. Lauderdale was Cozumel. This was our second time to visit this island and one of our favorite places. The streets are filled with vendors selling everything from jewelry and artwork to flavored tequilas. We found it necessary to sample strawberry tequila. Yum. Live music filled the air as we sauntered from shop to shop. The air was warm and humid with occasional light sprinkles adding to the humidity. Cozumel is apparently popular with all travelers as it was our longest stay in port. We docked at 9 am and sailed at 11 pm. Don and I enjoyed lunch at a little café called Kiss My Cactus. As we perused through one of the shops, the manager introduced himself and asked us about our white canes. He told us about his friend who was blind and his family would have nothing to do with him. He realized that the cane would be of help to his friend. We promised the manager that we would send a cane for his friend which we did upon arriving home.

We continued on purchasing gifts for friends and family and took a taxi back to the ship. After dinner on the ship, Don and I disembarked again and walked around the port area. It would be our final excursion before setting sail for Florida.

Dining on cruise ships is fine dining at its best. Food is available twenty-four hours a day and in numerous ship locations. I remember being told on my first cruise as I was objecting to the desserts being offered that I shouldn't worry. I was assured that it is the salt air that shrinks clothes. Dinner is always a multi-course event including several choices of appetizers, soups, salads, and always numerous choices for entrees and desserts. My favorite soups were the chilled ones, including blueberry melon and strawberry cream. My favorite dessert was the incredible chocolate soufflé.

Negotiating some parts of the ship could be challenging. The sleeping rooms, however, were numbered in Braille. The smaller numbers began at the bow of the ship and got bigger toward the fantail. Odd numbered rooms were on the starboard side of the ship and the even numbers were on the port side. This system made locating rooms quite easy for me.

If you're in the market for diamonds or gemstones, the Caribbean is the place to shop. Jewelry stores line the streets of nearly all of these islands. I must admit I have enjoyed spending some time browsing these shops and contributing to the local economy.

Don and I always enjoy walking around the outer decks of the ships. Our favorite spot to stop and spend some time was at the fantail. Standing at the back of the ship listening to the wake below is truly an awesome experience. As the powerful engines move the ship forward the sound of massive amounts of ocean water churning below us is a sound like none other. As the warm winds wrap around us and the ship sways gently over the azure blue ocean, we always realize our love of cruising and lament the fact that the trip is all too soon concluded.

I have now described to you in some detail one of my favorite vacations. If you are possibly one of those people who might ask me how I could enjoy traveling, perhaps this has helped to answer some of your questions.

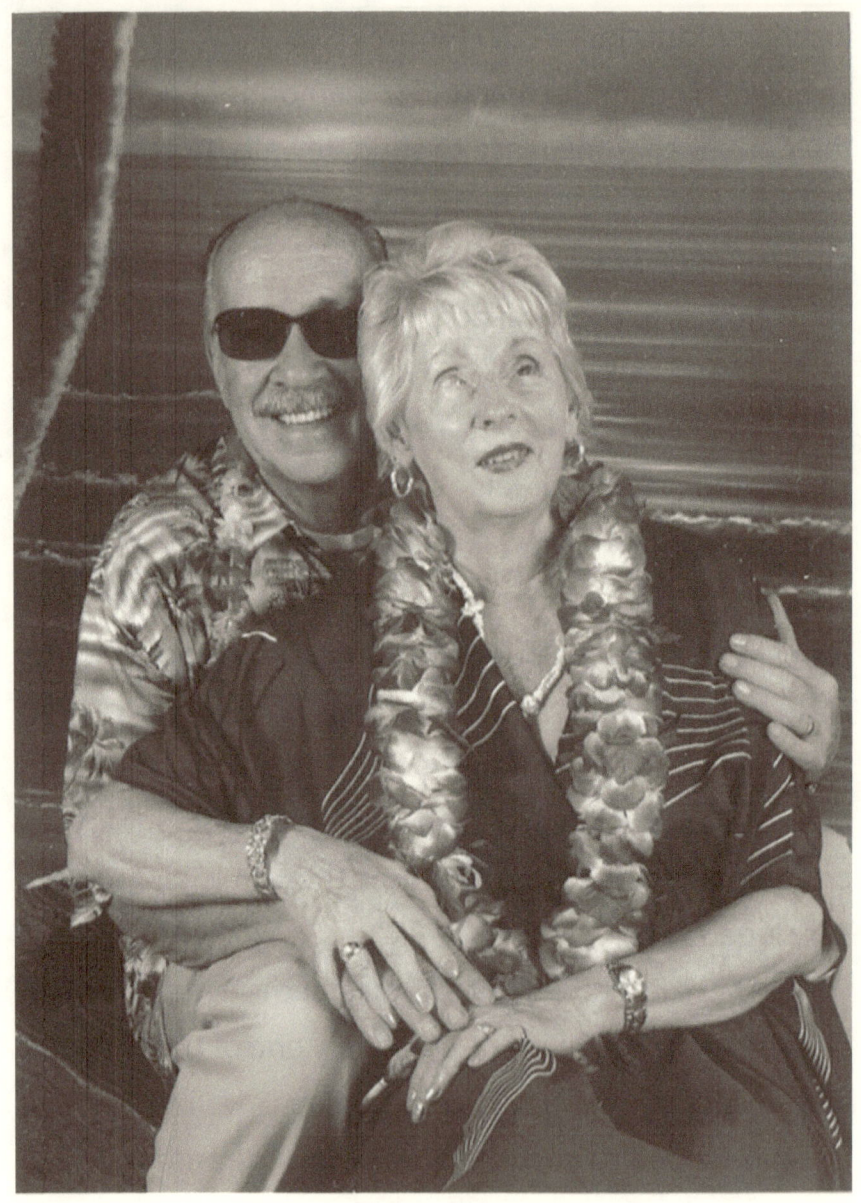

Anniversary Cruise to Hawaii

CHAPTER EIGHTEEN

My Spiritual Journey

This subject has been saved for the final chapter since it is an unfinished chapter. My awareness, my spirituality, and my philosophy of life, have been an ongoing journey. I consider myself a student of life, and I continue to learn each day.

This journey began in my childhood while living with my grandparents in a rural area of the Midwest. Grandma and Grandpa were hard-working, generous, loving, and religious people. They shared meals and worked closely with the neighbors. They attended church regularly and contributed in many ways to the community. My sister and I lived for many years with our grandparents. Our parents had divorced when I was seven years old and Janice was only a baby. We were not allowed to spend time with our dad. I have few memories of him but I believe he loved his little girls. I have heard stories that he would take me places to proudly show off his daughter.

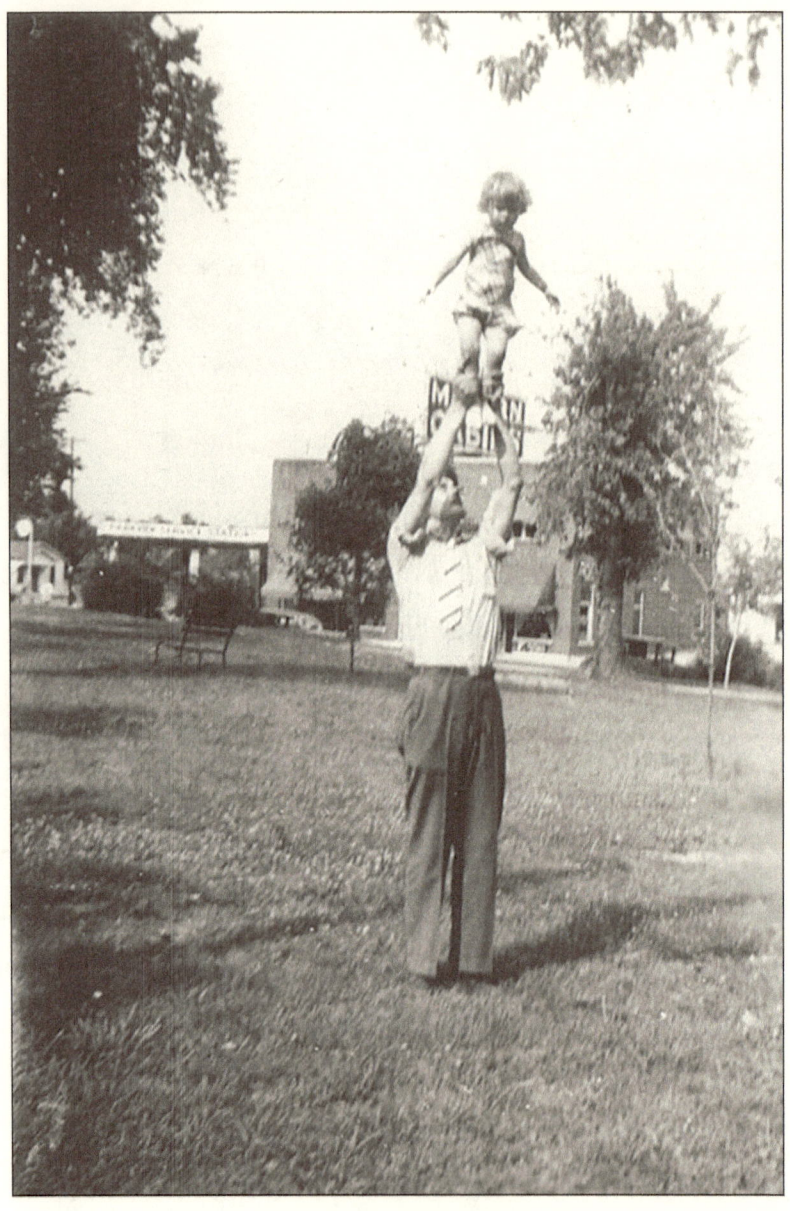

Nancy and Dad

Janice has no memories of her father as she was a tiny baby when she was taken to live with our grandparents. Our mother believed this was necessary because she was now a single, working parent and was unable to care for her children.

The doctrine our grandparents followed was tough, at least for me as a kid. Movies and card games (even the kid's kind) were frowned upon. To me, their God seemed harsh yet loving at the same time. I had difficulty with this contradiction. I often heard our preacher elaborate on how we would burn in hell if we sinned. On the other hand, some of my fondest memories are of my participation in church and Sunday school. I could recite the names of the books of the Bible from Genesis to Revelations. I memorized verses and even read aloud from my Braille Bible during church meetings. Christmas time was so very special with the singing of Christmas carols and the beautiful Christmas pageants. Church-organized picnics and hayrides were also fun for the Sunday school group.

When I left home, my contact with church was intermittent. I knew that I needed the connection, but there was still a part of religion I did not understand. For a while I called myself agnostic, feeling there was a Higher Power, but I wasn't clear on how to define that Higher Power.

When my boys were small, I attended a nearby

church and took them to Sunday school. I wanted them to have exposure to religion. I am sure I did not send any clear messages to them because of my own confusion about the subject. They have come to their own conclusion as adults, as has their mom.

While working on my Masters program, I returned to reading, both from necessity, as well as desire. I read and reread Mazlow, Jung, and Satir. I began reading the more recent motivational authors such as Chopra, Williamson, and Dyer. The more I read, the more I wanted to read. Access to these books has been made easier for me now that audible books are available at the local bookstores. There is now a wonderful variety of information readily available to me. I read about philosophers and saints and of healers and spiritual leaders. I have attempted to understand Einstein's theory of relativity and quantum physics. I have struggled with Milton's essay on blindness. On the lighter side, I also enjoy a romantic comedy and have spent hours browsing through some of my favorite cook books. With all of this, I have only scratched the surface, but this endeavor has brought about some insight and caused me to search my own soul for answers. This is not an attempt to convince anyone of anything. This is to encourage more reading, studying, and soul-searching. What I do believe is that religion or spirituality or whatever you prefer to call it, is an ongoing and evolving process. It is also my belief that through living our lives, and experiencing our experiences, comes growth, understanding, and opportunity. I know that any success I may have experienced has been a result of challenges I have previously encountered. There has been a lesson to learn in every problem I have resolved.

Adversity is one of life's greatest teachers. In addition to this, the people we find the most difficult to work with are our greatest instructors. This was personally a bitter pill for me to swallow on more than one occasion. However, these difficult people have taught me how not to live my life. These lessons have been bittersweet, but they have been lessons worth learning.

I am happy to report that I have found a church that meets my needs, and I have learned that God, or the Higher Power, is all about love. The more love you give away, the more you will have to give. It seems so simple, but is not always that easy to do. I am reminded of Mother Theresa's comments when she was asked how she was able to love and nurture the sick on the streets of Calcutta. She said that she saw the face of Jesus in every single person. It's a tough call to even attempt to live up to the standards of Mother Theresa, but the world needs more love, more compassion, and more understanding. Whether we are working with a terminally ill patient, or our next door neighbor, let us lead with kindness and generosity. Let us share love and compassion. Let us not judge.

During my life experiences and my growth processes, I have given much credit to my mentors who counseled and guided me through problems and taught me to be confident, even as a blind person. I now understand that these people did not appear in my life coincidentally— there are no coincidences. There is a reason for everything. My Higher Power, my God, has carefully put me in contact with the right people at the right time. These people reached into their souls and shared with me generously of their knowledge and wisdom. It is the least I can do to reach into my soul and pass this love and concern on to others. This is what life is all about.

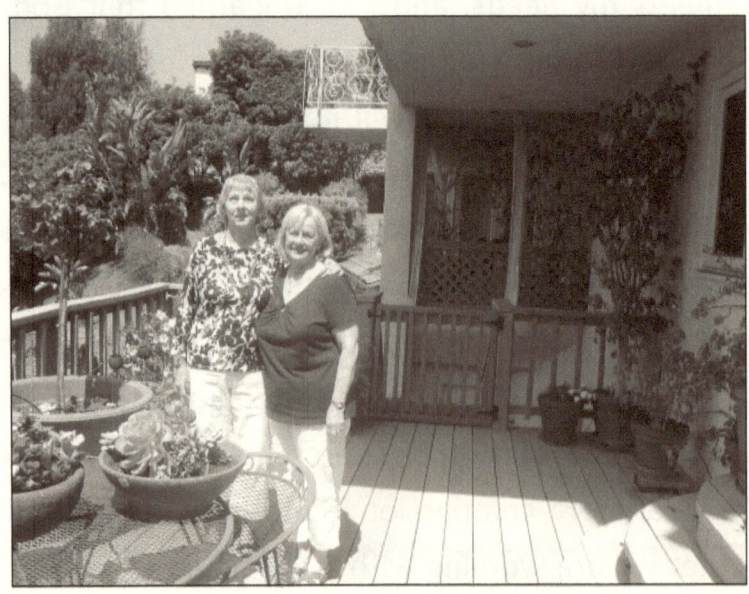

Hanging out with my Sister

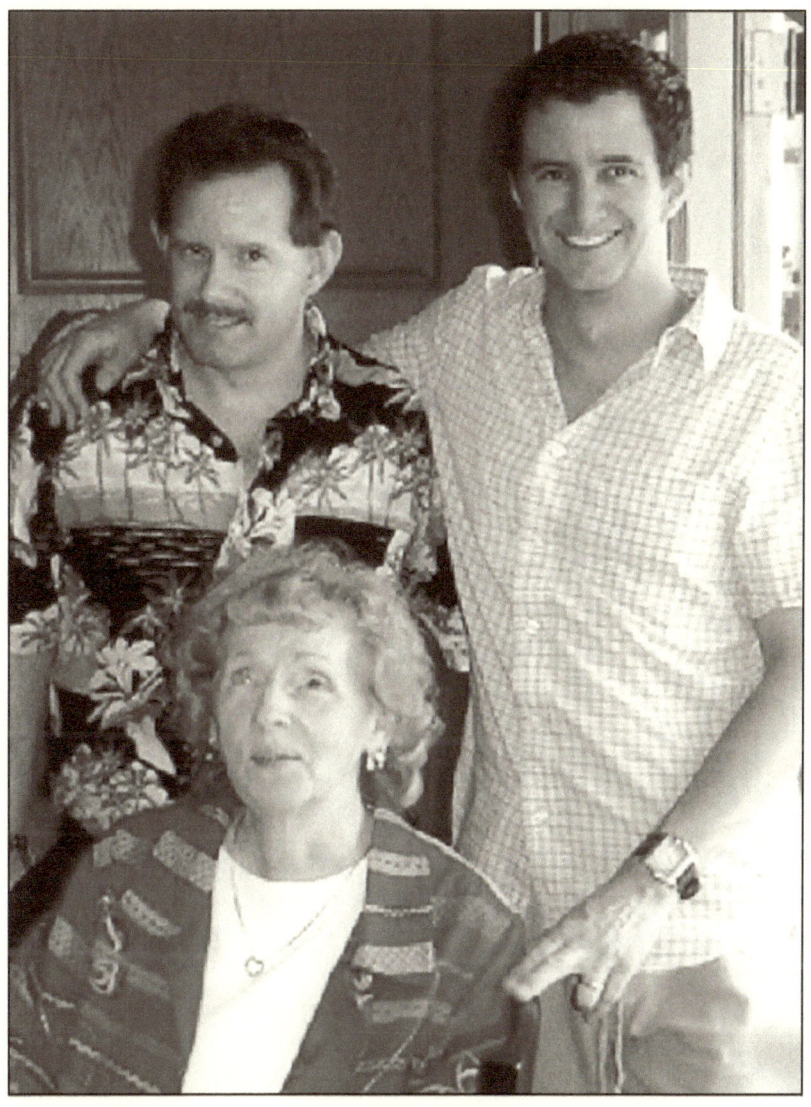

My Two Sons

ACKNOWLEDGMENTS

My loving husband, Don, for his ongoing support

My son, Jeff, for building my new computer

My son, Kevin, for his insightful contributions

My patient sister, Janice, for searching through stacks of family photos

Louise Kodituwakku for her professional input on one of my most difficult chapters to write

Nancy Levine for her guidance and her belief in my ability

Pastor David Snyman for his input and encouragement

Rhonda Arkana, Patty Kuning and Amy Schreiber for their computer expertise.

----------------- E N D N O T E S :-----------------

1 *Walking Alone and Marching Together: A History of the Organized Blind Movement in the United States, 1940-1990*, by Floyd Matson. P. 14, ..."Collectively, we are the masters of our own future and the successful guardian of our own common interests.", proclaimed Dr. Jacobus tenBroek.

2 Americans with Disabilities Act, 1990, http://www.ada.gov/pubs/ada.htm.

3 Correspondence from the Missouri School for the Blind.

4 Retinitis pigmentosa is an eye disease characterized by the slow decrease in peripheral vision.

5 NFBC Journal, Fall/Winter 2005, President's Report (available through Jacobus tenBroek library NFB), www.nfb.org,

6 NFBC Journal, Spring/Summer 2003, "Braille is Beautiful Workshop", by Nancy Burns.

7 Other organizations serving the blind or visually impaired community include, but are not limited to, the following: American Foundation for the Blind, http://www.afb.org/ Braille Institute of America, http://www.brailleinstitute.org/ National Federation of the Blind, http://www.nfb.org

8 Macular degeneration is a medical condition usually of older adults which results in a loss of vision in the center of the visual field.

9 AB2326, (2006) Braille Reading and Math Standards, California Department of Education, Braille Reading Standards, p. viii, http://www.cde.ca.gov/sp/se/sr/documents/braillereadstand.pdf. The section entitled "Braille Bias" was written by this author.

www.ingramcontent.com/pod-product-compliance
Lightning Source LLC
Chambersburg PA
CBHW020257290526
45784CB00003B/1279